Respiratory Care:
Assessment and management

Full the full range of M&K Publishing books please visit our website:
www.mkupdate.co.uk

Respiratory Care:
Assessment and management

Deborah Duncan

Respiratory Care: Assessment and management

Deborah Duncan

ISBN: 978-1-910451-02-1

First published 2017

British Library Cataloguing in Publication Data

A catalogue record for this book is available from the British Library

Notice

Clinical practice and medical knowledge constantly evolve. Standard safety precautions must be followed, but, as knowledge is broadened by research, changes in practice, treatment and drug therapy may become necessary or appropriate. Readers must check the most current product information provided by the manufacturer of each drug to be administered and verify the dosages and correct administration, as well as contraindications. It is the responsibility of the practitioner, utilising the experience and knowledge of the patient, to determine dosages and the best treatment for each individual patient. Any brands mentioned in this book are as examples only and are not endorsed by the publisher. Neither the publisher nor the authors assume any liability for any injury and/or damage to persons or property arising from this publication.

To contact M&K Publishing write to:

M&K Update Ltd · The Old Bakery · St. John's Street

Keswick · Cumbria CA12 5AS

Tel: 01768 773030 · Fax: 01768 781099

publishing@mkupdate.co.uk

www.mkupdate.co.uk

Designed and typeset by Mary Blood

Printed in England by H&H Reeds, Penrith

Contents

List of figures vi

List of tables vi

List of boxes vi

About the author viii

List of abbreviations ix

Introduction xi

Acknowledgements xii

Chapter 1: A quick look at anatomy and physiology 1

Chapter 2: Respiratory assessment 15

Chapter 3: Physical assessment 29

Chapter 4: Secondary data 37

Chapter 5: Acute conditions 47

Chapter 6: Chronic conditions 59

Chapter 7: Self-management 85

Chapter 8: Pharmacology 95

Chapter 9: Intermediate, home-based and end of life care 107

Glossary 113

Index 126

List of figures

Figure 1.1: Diagram of the lungs 5
Figure 1.2: Cellular respiration 6
Figure 1.3: A summary of gas transport and exchange 9
Figure 2.1: Example of a genogram 19
Figure 3.1: The anatomical landmarks of the chest 29
Figure 4.1: Flow graphs 43
Figure 6.1: Asthma and the airways 66
Figure 6.2: Stepwise asthma management 71

List of tables

Table 1.1: Muscles involved in breathing 5
Table 2.1: MRCP scale 16
Table 2.2: Work-related diseases 20
Table 2.3: Causes of cough 22
Table 2.4: Specific areas to consider, relating to respiratory disease 25
Table 3.1: Breathe sounds 33
Table 3.2: Adventitious abnormal sounds 34
Table 3.3: Respiratory chest examination checklist 35
Table 4.1: Specific tests 37
Table 4.2: Full blood count results 39
Table 4.3: Severity of airflow obstruction 43
Table 6.1: The '3 questions' screening tool 69
Table 6.2: PAINT 74
Table 7.1: Factors affecting medical adherence 87

List of boxes

Box 1.1:   Cystic fibrosis 3
Box 1.2:   Hypercapnia 8
Box 1.3a: Reader activity 11
Box 1.3b: Answers to reader activity 12
Box 2.1:   The components of history taking 16
Box 2.2:   The HOPE questionnaire 20
Box 2.3a: Reader activity 21
Box 2.4a: Reader activity 24
Box 2.3b: Answers to reader activity 26

Box 2.4b: Answers to reader activity 26

Box 4.1:   The Bode method 45

Box 4.2:   The approximate 4-year survival interpretation 45

Box 5.1:   CURB65 score for mortality risk assessment 51

Box 5.2:   Signs and symptoms of hypercapnia 55

Box 6.1:   Presentation of COPD 60

Box 6.2:   Reader activity 64

Box 6.3:   Diagnosis and the probability of asthma in children 68

Box 6.4:   Asthma triggers 72

Box 6.5a: Reader activity – case study 73

Box 6.5b: Answers to reader activity 80

Box 7.1a: Reader activity 85

Box 7.1b: Answers to reader activity 91

Box 8.1:   Inhaled drugs commonly used in respiratory disease 95

Box 8.2a: Reader activity 96

Box 8.2b: Answers to reader activity 103

About the author

Deborah Duncan BSc PGCAP PGDIP MSc FHEA AKC RGN RM MP NT
Senior Lecturer in Adult Nursing, Bucks New University
and Associate Lecturer, Kings College London

Deborah is an experienced lecturer for pre-qualification and post-registration nursing students and is involved in developing e-learning courses for nurses. She is also an advanced nurse practitioner with 17 years experience in primary care, and diagnosing and managing patients with long-term conditions. She is also a member of the association of respiratory nurse specialists.

Although this is her first text book she is a prolific writer, having had over thirty articles published in the nursing press, and has written two non-nursing books to date, one of which is a novel.

List of abbreviations

Explanations of most of these abbreviations can be found in the glossary at the back of the book.

2MWT 2-Minute Walk Test

ACOS Asthma—Chronic Obstructive Pulmonary Disease Overlap Syndrome

A1AT alpha 1-antitrypsin

ABG arterial blood gas

ACE angiotensin-converting enzyme

ACOS Asthma—Chronic Obstructive Pulmonary Disease Overlap Syndrome

ALS amyotrophic lateral sclerosis

ANCA antineutrophil cytoplasmic antibody

APC antigen presenting cell

ASL airway surface liquid

ATP adenosine triphosphate

BAL bronchoscopic alveolar lavage

BDP beclometasone dipropionate

BMI body mass index

BLVR bronchoscopic lung volume reduction

COPD chronic obstructive pulmonary disease

CRP C-reactive protein

CT computed tomography

ECG electrocardiogram

ESR erythrocyte sedimentation rate

FBC full blood count

FEV1 forced expiratory volume in one second

FVC forced vital capacity

GCM gene complex molecule

GORD gastric-oesophageal reflux disease

g/dL grams per decilitre

HaH hospital at home

Hb haemoglobin

HRQOL health-related quality of life

HVS hyperventilation syndrome

IHC inhaled corticosteroid

INR international normalised ratio blood test

IV intravenous

JVP jugular venous pressure

LABA long-acting beta2 agonist

LAMA long-acting muscarinic antagonist

LDH lactate dehydrogenase

LHF left-handed heart failure

LTOT long-term oxygen therapy

LVF left ventricular failure

LVRS lung volume reduction surgery

MCH mean cell haemoglobin

MCV mean corpuscular volume

MDI metered dose inhaler

MHC major histocompatibility complex

mmHg millimetres of mercury (Hg)

NSAID non-steroidal anti-inflammatory drug

NSCLC non-small cell carcinoma

PaO$_2$ partial pressure of oxygen

PaCO$_2$ partial pressure of carbon dioxide

PCV packed cell volume

RAST radioallergosorbent

SABA short-acting beta2 agonist

SAMA short-acting muscarinic antagonist

SLE systemic lupus erythematosus

μmol micromole (a unit of measurement)

Introduction

This textbook is written for health professionals caring for patients with a respiratory condition. There are a great many respiratory conditions so the book will look at the most common ones. More than 30% of patients who visit a general practitioner each year have a respiratory condition (Fischer *et al.* 2005, Van Dujin *et al.* 2007). The most common types of problems are uncomplicated upper respiratory tract infections (the common cold) and bronchitis (Fischer *et al.* 2005).

This book will look at both acute and chronic conditions. Respiratory conditions are also categorised according to whether they are restrictive or obstructive. An obstructive disease causes damage to the lung tissue or narrowing in the airways. A patient may inhale but struggle to exhale effectively, causing a feeling of breathlessness. Common examples of obstructive conditions are chronic obstructive pulmonary disease (COPD) and asthma. People with restrictive lung disease cannot fully fill their lungs, as their lungs are restricted from doing so. Common examples of restrictive disorders are interstitial lung disease (such as idiopathic pulmonary fibrosis) and hypoventilation syndrome.

The first chapter gives the reader an overview of the respiratory system. Several chapters then look at history taking, and the physical assessment and secondary tests you need to do to assess a patient with an undiagnosed respiratory condition. We will also look at the aetiology, assessment and management of specific conditions, followed by a chapter on the pharmacology of respiratory disease. Finally, we look at intermediate, hospital at home and end of life care.

This book offers a holistic and practical approach to caring for a patient with a respiratory disease. Most of the chapters also include at least one reader activity as well as a list of further resources. For easy reference, there is a list of abbreviations on p. ix and a glossary on p. 113.

References

Fischer, T., Fischer, S., Kochen, M.M. & Hummers-Pradier, E. (2005). Influence of patient symptoms and physical findings on general practitioners' treatment of respiratory tract infections: a direct observation study. *BMC Family Practice*. **6**(1), 1.

Van Dujin, H., Kuyvenhoven, M., Schellevis, F. & Verheij, T (2007). Illness behaviour and antibiotic prescription in patients with respiratory tract symptoms. *Journal of General Practice*. **57**(540), 561–68.

Acknowledgements

My thanks and acknowledgements go to Dr Carole Jackson, Julie Bliss, Alison Gallagher and my colleagues at The Florence Nightingale Faculty of Nursing and Midwifery, who supported me while I planned this book. Also to those at Bucks New University – thank you for welcoming me.

Thanks also go to my friends and family, particularly my husband Malcolm, who supported me while I wrote it.

Chapter 1

A quick look at anatomy and physiology

To assess and manage a patient with a respiratory problem, you need to have a full understanding of the anatomy and physiology of that system. This chapter will discuss the role of the respiratory system, concentrating on its major anatomical structures. It will then look at the science of respiration. There is also a reader activity at the end of the chapter.

The respiratory system

The respiratory system carries out the activity of breathing or inhalation. This is the movement of air into the lungs to supply the body with oxygen. The respiratory system is also responsible for the movement of air out of the **lungs**, to expel carbon dioxide, known as exhalation.

The major anatomical structures in the respiratory system are: the nose, **pharynx**, **larynx**, **trachea**, the two **bronchi** and the lungs. The lungs include the bronchioles and the alveoli. The lungs themselves are surrounded by the **pleurae**. There is a thin layer of tissue called the visceral pleura, which covers the lungs. This layer also covers the chest wall and surrounds the heart and is called the parietal pleura. There is a thin layer of fluid between the visceral and parietal pleurae, which allows movement between them. The space between the visceral and parietal layers is called the **pleural space**.

The respiratory system is divided into two parts. One is the conducting part, which passes air into the lungs. This includes the nasal passages and the pharynx, larynx, trachea, bronchi and larger bronchioles. The second part is called the respiratory part, and this is where gas exchange occurs in the smaller bronchioles and alveoli.

The nose is the start of the respiratory system. The **nasal cavity** is hollow so the air passes through it, while being heated and moistened. The cavity is lined with hair and **mucus**, which acts a filter, trapping foreign particles. The other opening is the mouth or oval cavity. The nose is generally used for the activity of breathing, as the mouth lacks a filter system. This explains why people who breathe through their mouths have a higher incidence of oral infections (Abreu et al. 2008, Gulati, Grewal & Kaur 1998). The air is then passed to the pharynx.

The pharynx is a fibromuscular tube situated behind the nasal cavity, the oral cavity and the larynx. It is usually called the throat and extends from the base of the skull level to **C6** or the **cricoid**

cartilage. Its function is to deliver food products from the mouth to the **oesophagus**. It also warms, moistens and filters the air we inhale.

The **nasopharynx** is found behind the nasal cavity and the **soft palate**. When you swallow food, it passes through the **oropharynx** and the **laryngopharynx**. The soft palate rises, allowing the pharyngeal wall to pull forward and form a seal over the nasopharynx. The oropharynx lies between the soft palate and the base of the tongue. The narrower laryngopharynx extends from the **hyoid bone** and the start of the oesophagus.

The two laryngeal cartilages that can be felt during a neck examination are the laryngeal cartilage (or 'Adam's apple') and the slightly lower cricoid cartilage. The distance between the laryngeal cartilage and the **sternal notch** is used to assess lung hyperinflation (Bickley 2003).

The warmed air then leaves the pharynx and enters the larynx (voice box). This is an area of ligaments and muscle. The trachea is attached to the cricoid cartilage of the larynx. It is roughly 2.5cm in diameter and 10–12cm long. The walls are surrounded by cartilage to protect the airway from collapsing. In the disorder **tracheomalacia**, there can be a weakness in the longitudinal fibres of the trachea or impaired cartilage integrity which can cause trapping and collection of secretions that can lead to infection (Carden *et al*. 2005). Interestingly the shape of the adult trachea varies even without disease – as some remain circular and others a more ovoid shape (Tewfik & Gest 2015).

The trachea divides into the right and left main bronchi at the keel-like partition called the **carina**. It is situated to the left of the median line. However, the right bronchus appears to be more central than the left, making it look like a direct continuation of the trachea (Tewfik & Gest 2015). It then branches into the lobar, segmental and sub-segmental bronchi. It divides a further 25 times into the pulmonary alveoli at the terminal ends of the respiratory tree where the gas transfer occurs.

The first seven divisions are called the larger airways. These contain:

- **Ciliated epithelium**, which contains **goblet cells**. These glandular cells secrete a gel-forming mucin found in mucus, called **airway surface liquid** (**ASL**). ASL has a mucus component that traps the inhaled particles and a soluble layer, which keeps mucus at an optimum distance from the underlying epithelia, preventing easy clearance (Tarran 2004).
- Mucus-secreting cells in the submucosal.
- **Endocrine** cells.
- Cartilage and smooth muscle in the branch walls.

The remaining 16–18 branches are called the **small airways**. They have cells that produce **surfactant**, which reduces the surface tension of fluid in the lungs. They contain fewer goblet cells and there is no cartilage present.

Box 1.1: Cystic fibrosis

In the genetic disorder **cystic fibrosis**, the goblet cells in the mucosal produce thick, sticky mucus. It cannot be transported out of the respiratory system by the **cilia** that line the tract. The smaller passages become blocked with this dense mucus, leading to significant infection and poor gas exchange.

Air flow

The movement of air in the respiratory system depends on the difference in air pressure between the oral cavity and the pulmonary alveoli. When you breathe in, the **intrathoracic pressure** drops below the **atmospheric pressure**. The air is therefore forced into the alveolar tree. When you breathe out, the muscles in the lung and chest wall recoil like elastic. This causes the intrathoracic pressure to rise above atmospheric pressure. In Alpha-1 antitrypsin (A1AT) deficiency there is a lack of the elasticity needed to allow the airways to recoil.

The rate at which air can move along the airways therefore depends on any resistance in the airway. Any problem with the **lumen** of the airway can potentially increase this resistance. Such problems can include:

- Contents blocking the lumen of the airway
- Internal or external pressure
- Lack of muscle tone
- The thickness of the epithelial lining.

Obstruction within the airways can be due to **smooth muscle spasm**, as in **asthma** and **chronic obstructive pulmonary disorder** (**COPD**), increased airways secretions or **sputum**.

The alveoli

There are over 150 million small air-filled sacs in each lung. These are the alveoli, which are the terminal ends of the bronchi tree at the end of the bronchioles. Each alveolus contains type 1 and II alveolar cells, which have a thin cell wall to facilitate gas exchange. Type 1 is mainly a squamous cell; type II has a secretory function, producing surfactant. Each alveolus has a complicated network of hundreds of **capillaries**. These also have a thin membrane, facilitating gas exchange at the large alveolar capillary interface or membrane.

Lobes of the lungs

There are two lungs in the thoracic cavity. The right lung has three lobes, while the left lung has two lobes. This is important to remember when performing a physical assessment.

The respiratory muscles

The inspiratory muscles consist of three types of muscle. They are:

- The diaphragm
- The intercostal muscles
- The accessory muscles.

The diaphragm

The diaphragm is a dome-shaped muscle at the bottom of the lungs that separates the thoracic cavity from the abdominal pelvic cavity. It consists of two parts: the peripheral muscle which has radial muscle fibres extending from the ribs, sternum and the spinal column; and the central tendon. The central tendon is situated behind the **xiphisternal joint** and extends from ribs 4–7 and the anterior surface of the **lumbar vertebrae**. Being made of dense **collagen** fibres, it is a strong insertion point for the muscles.

When you inhale air into your lungs, the muscles in the diaphragm contract and pull the central tendon into the abdominal cavity. This allows the space within the thorax to increase, allowing more room for the air-filled lungs. You can feel this if you take a deep breath in, and place your hands on your abdomen.

The intercostal muscles

The intercostal muscles consist of the external and intercostal groups of muscles that run between the ribs and help form and move the chest wall. The external muscles start at the inferior border of each rib, and their role is to elevate the rib during inspiration. The internal muscles start at the superior border of each rib, and their role is to depress the ribs after exhalation.

The accessory muscles

The accessory muscles are found in the neck and shoulder area. These include: the sternomastoid, scalenus anterior, medius and posterior, pectoralis major and minor, inferior fibres of serratus anterior and latissimus dorsi, serratus posterior anterior and the iliocostalis cervicis muscles. They are mainly used for inspiration if a patient is having difficulty inhaling oxygen into the lung using the usual muscles of respiration.

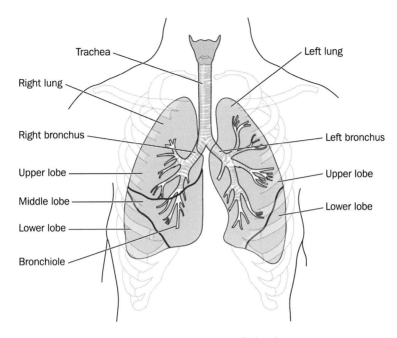

Figure 1.1: Diagram of the lungs

Males tend to use their diaphragms for breathing, whereas women tend to have greater thoracic movement.

Table 1.1: Muscles involved in breathing

Type of movement	Effect of the muscles	Muscles used
Quiet inspirational breathing	Increases the anterior posterior (AP) diameter Increases vertical diameter Increases transverse diameter	Diaphragm Scalenus muscles Upper intercostal muscles
Forced inspiration	Increases diameters	Diaphragm Scalenus muscles Sternocleidomastoid muscles Quadratus lumborum Erector spinae
Quiet expiration	Decreases all diameters	Recoil of the lungs Relaxation of diaphragm and intercostal muscles
Forced expiration	Decreases all diameters	Contraction of anterior abdominal wall muscles Diaphragm Intercostal muscles

The main function of the respiratory system

The main function of the lungs is to take oxygen from the air we inhale, and to exhale carbon dioxide. The air we breathe in (external respiration) is a mixture of gases, including nitrogen (N_2) and oxygen (O_2). Each gas contributes a partial pressure to become part of an atmospheric pressure of 760mmHg. The partial pressure of oxygen (PaO_2) is 20.9% of the total atmospheric pressure. This decreases to 13.2% as the air passes through the warmed respiratory tract, across the respiratory membrane, into the alveoli in the lungs. The gases then diffuse into the pulmonary capillaries. The result is that the PaO_2 levels in the bloodstream rise and the $PaCO_2$ levels fall.

Internal respiration is the term used to describe this process, as the gases are diffused between the blood and interstitial fluid and the capillary cell membranes.

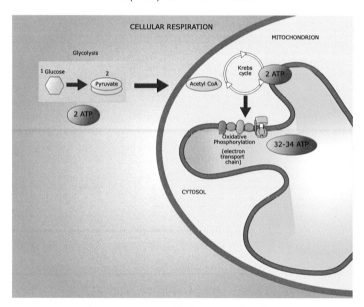

Figure 1.2: Cellular respiration

The process of respiration

Several functions are required to achieve respiration. To enable the lungs to take oxygen from the air we inhale and to exhale carbon dioxide:

- The respiratory centre in the brain must regulate our speed and depth of breathing.
- The muscles in the chest have to enable us to inflate or deflate the lungs.
- The alveoli and capillaries in the lungs must transport oxygen and carbon dioxide.
- The pulmonary circulation has to move blood in and out of the lungs.
- Our immune system has to protect us against foreign particles.

Local control of respiration

The rate at which oxygen is delivered to the cellular tissue is regulated at a local level. Cells have a continuous need for oxygen, as they need to use the oxidative phosphorylation to generate their energy source known as adenosine triphosphate (ATP) (Pittman 2011). The cells also have an inbuilt ability to continuously monitor their metabolic requirements (Clanton, Hogan & Gladden 2013).

When the normal O_2 uptake and delivery changes, the cells have an elaborate and diverse sensing and response system to compensate for the alteration. If the peripheral tissue becomes more active, the interstitial PaO_2 drops and the levels of $PaCO_2$ rise in response. The partial pressures in the tissue are altered, resulting in more oxygen being delivered to the tissue. The smooth muscles in the arteriole walls relax to aid this process. When $PaCO_2$ levels increase, the bronchioles dilate, directing more O_2 to the areas that require it.

Control of breathing

The activity of breathing relies on the following anatomical structures:

- The respiratory centre in the brain
- The spinal cord
- The nerves
- The neuromuscular junctions
- The pleurae
- The lungs
- The muscles
- The chest wall
- The **anterior horn cells**.

The respiratory centre in the brain controls the involuntary component of breathing. Groups of dorsal **neurons** are based in the **medulla oblongata** and **pons** of the **brainstem**. These regulate the respiratory muscles and therefore control the frequency (rate) and depth of breathing. The dorsal neurons generate repetitive respiratory signals which build up over 2 seconds and result in the smooth contraction of the respiratory muscles. After inspiration, there is a 3-second time lag, allowing the muscles to relax and expiration to occur. The process then repeats itself. The cycle takes a total of 5 seconds.

The normal respiratory rate is therefore 12 respirations per minute.

The brain also detects any changes via **sensory receptors** such as the partial pressure of oxygen and carbon dioxide, or via **mechanoreceptors** in the stretch and relaxation of the muscles. The mechanoreceptors respond to any change to the volume of the lungs or the arterial blood pressure.

The **baroreceptors** are free nerve endings situated in the elastic tissue of the blood vessels. When the pressure changes the blood vessel wall contracts or dilates. The baroreceptors react immediately to this pressure. They are found in the **carotid artery** and the **aorta**.

There are chemoreceptors in the carotid and aorta arteries which monitor the oxygen and carbon dioxide concentration of the blood and the pH of the blood. When these levels drop, neuro-signals are sent to the brain via the **glossopharyngeal** and **vagal nerves**. They respond much more sensitively to an increase of $PaCO_2$. If there is a small increase in CO_2 levels such as 0.13kPa, there can be an increase of 2−4L/min in ventilation. If increased levels of $PaCO_2$ persist, the chemoreceptors become less sensitive to these changes. This can be seen in patients with **hypercapnia**.

Cellular respiration produces carbon dioxide as a waste product. The cells remove the CO_2 from the tissues by means of hydration to a **bicarbonate ion**. This ion is carried to the lungs via the blood **plasma**, where it is converted back into CO_2 and released during exhalation.

While it is in the blood, the bicarbonate ion also neutralises acid introduced to the blood through other metabolic processes (such as during exercise, when lactic acid is produced).

The **bicarbonate buffering system** also works with the lungs through respiratory compensation. In respiratory compensation, the pH of the blood plasma can be altered by varying the respiratory rate. Receptors are stimulated by an increase in hydrogen ions – as in the case of metabolic **alkalosis** or diabetic **acidosis**.

The normal pH of the blood is 7.35. **Acidaemia** is defined as a pH < 7.35. **Alkalaemia** is defined as a pH > 7.45.

To keep the pH stable, the ratio of bicarbonate to carbonic acid must always be 20:1. The **homeostasis** is mainly maintained by the respiratory and renal systems. In the renal system, the kidneys regulate the concentration of the bicarbonate ion by filtering out excess amounts or by retaining it when it is only present in low concentrations.

The bicarbonate buffering system is one mechanism that maintains a neutral pH in the blood. Homeostasis involves the balance of carbonic acid (H_2CO_3), bicarbonate ion (HCO_3^-), and carbon dioxide (CO_2) in order to maintain the pH in the blood and duodenum. Carbon dioxide is **catalysed** by the enzyme carbonic anhydrase and reacts with water (H_2O) to form carbonic acid (H_2CO_3). This then forms a hydrogen ion and bicarbonate ion.

$$CO_2 + H_2O \rightleftharpoons H_2CO_3 \rightleftharpoons HCO_3^- + H_3O^+$$

Box 1.2: Hypercapnia

The prefix 'hyper' comes from the Greek word meaning 'too much'. In hypercapnia, there is an increase in $PaCO_2$ in the arterial blood. When this change is identified by the chemoreceptors in the carotid and aortic vessels, the respiratory centre is stimulated to increase ventilation. The result is hyperventilation, meaning an increase in the rate and depth of respiration. There is also an increase in the transportation of carbon dioxide from the capillaries back out through the lungs.

Oxygen transportation

Arterial blood only contains 1.5% of free oxygen molecules. The majority of oxygen molecules are bound to the iron ions in **haemoglobin** (**Hb**) molecules. The amount of oxygen bound to the haemoglobin in the cell depends on the surrounding partial O_2. The percentage of O_2 in the haemoglobin in the blood vessels leaving the lungs is approximately 95−100%. This high percentage makes the arterial blood bright red in colour. It can drop to 70%, once the blood has been transported to the waiting cell membranes, which explains why venous blood can appear to be a purple colour.

The Hb level in your blood can be assessed with a blood test. Normal Hb results can vary from person to person. They are in the following ranges:

Male: 13.8−17.2g/dL.

Female: 12.1−15.1g/dL

The result may also be written as grams per litre (g/L) depending on the laboratory used.

Oxygen saturation in the blood

The colour of blood is determined by the amount of haemoglobin in the blood. A patient can appear 'blue' or cyanotic at their extremities or mucous membranes, such as the mouth. This can help us estimate the amount of oxygen in the blood, using pulse oximetry.

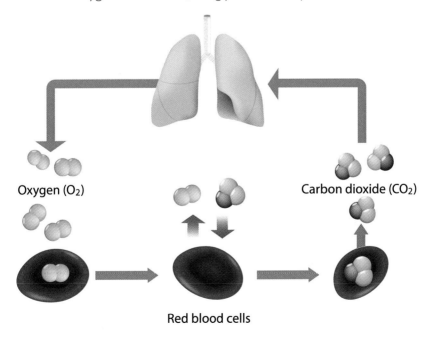

Oxygen (O_2)

Carbon dioxide (CO_2)

Red blood cells

Figure 1.3: A summary of gas transport and exchange

The defence of the respiratory system

The body has a range of systems that defend the lung tissue against inhaled foreign particles. Adults can inhale 10,000L of air in a day, which can contain a range of allergens, organisms and pollutants (Tomashefsk 2008).

To prevent the foreign particles reaching the lungs, the nasal hairs trap larger particles, which can be blown or sneezed away later. Particles smaller than $2-10\mu$mol are trapped in the sticky mucus produced by the barrier cells which line the length of the airways (Tomashefsk 2008). The mucus can be removed by the **mucociliary escalator** (Oberdörster 1988). This is often described as a 'conveyor belt', which moves the trapped particles and mucus. The beating cilia propel the trapped particles and gel that line the airways into the pharynx.

Coughing or sneezing can occur if receptors detect the presence of foreign particles. The muscle layer contracts, causing **bronchospasm**, which aids removal of the particle.

If they reach the alveoli, they are trapped and left in the alveoli fluid. Patients that have recurrent infections can have a bronchoscopic lung washout and these tiny particles can be tested under **microscopy**. There are also **macrophages** that surround the alveoli and can engulf any foreign visitors.

Innate and adaptive immunity

Innate immunity is a non-specific immune response to foreign particles. This is the first response to any invader. The **airway surface liquid** (**ASL**) contains several proteins which have microbial activity, responding to an alteration in the pH or salt concentration. Mediators are also released, such as lactoferrin, lysozyme, collectins and defensins, which are in turn activated. This activation results in the **lysis** of **pathogens**, or their destruction by rapidly adaptive immune cells such as **phagocytes** that dispose of the foreign particle. The major constituent of ASL is lysozyme, which is particularly sensitive to **gram-positive bacteria** such as *Haemophilus influenzae*, *Klebsiella pneumoniae* and *Escherichia coli*.

Adaptive immunity

The adaptive immune response within the respiratory system involves the production of neutralising **antibodies** and **T-lymphocytes**. However, the T-lymphocytes can alter the fine balance between clearing the pathogen and tissue damage, due to the **cytokines** that are secreted during this process (Boyton & Openshaw 2002).

There are four types of 'memory cells' that respond to specific **antigens** within the respiratory system. The response time to identify and destroy them varies in each case.

1. **Antigen-presenting cells** (**APCs**): The **dendritic cells** are one of the three types of APCs and they are very efficient at internalising antigens. They do this by means of **phagocytosis** or by receptor-mediated **endocytosis**, engulfing the pathogen. The dendritic cells head to the

lymphatic system, while processing the antigens from the cell wall of the organism. They then carry a fragment of the antigen-bound **major histocompatibility complex** (**MHC**) on their cell membrane. The MHC is a group of genes that encodes the cell surface molecules. The T-lymphocyte then recognises the encoded gene complex molecule (GCM).

2. CD4+ cells: These white blood cells are part of the human immune system and they work with the T-lymphocyte receptor. Their main role is to relay signals to other types of immune cells by recruiting the enzyme tyrosine kinase lymphocyte-specific protein. This is needed to activate other cells (such as the **CD8 cells**), which then destroy the pathogen.

3. Th1 response: When the T-lymphocyte recognises the antigen on an antigen-presenting cell, the **TCR-CD3** complex binds strongly to the MHC complex present on the surface of professional APCs. This stimulates the intracellular kinases present on cell proteins to activate major T-lymphocyte intracellular pathways. These active pathways are known as Signal 1 of T-lymphocyte activation.

4. Th2 response occurs when a T-lymphocyte has a further encounter with a specific antigen. These 'memory T-lymphocytes' (also known as 'antigen-experienced T cells') are re-activated using the same TCR pathways outlined above.

Do the following activity to see how much you remember about what has been discussed in this chapter.

Box 1.3a: Reader activity

1. Define what is meant by external and internal respiration.
2. Identify where the brainstem is found, and where the respiratory centre is located.
3. What colours the blood?
4. Name the respiratory muscles.

Summary

Understanding the anatomy and physiology of the respiratory system helps to inform you of where things can go wrong. You will develop a clearer understanding of the different disease processes that affect this system, and this in turn will help you make informed decisions when diagnosing and managing respiratory disease.

Box 1.3b: Answers to reader activity

1. Define what is meant by external and internal respiration.

In external respiration, oxygen is diffused into the blood, and carbon dioxide is diffused into the alveolar air. This exchange of gases occurs in the lungs. Internal respiration occurs in the tissues, rather than the lungs. In this process, oxygen diffuses out of the blood and carbon dioxide diffuses out of the cells.

2. Identify where the brainstem is found, and where the respiratory centre is located.

The brainstem is the region of the brain that connects the cerebrum with the spinal cord. The dorsal neurons that control breathing are found in the medulla oblongata and the pons.

3. What colours the blood?

The blood is red in colour because of the iron in the haemoglobin. Venous blood is much darker than arterial blood because oxygenated (arterial) blood is 'redder' than deoxygenated blood.

4. Name the respiratory muscles.

The respiratory muscles are the diaphragm and the intercostal and accessory muscles.

References

Abreu, R.R., Rocha, R.L., Lamounier, J.A. & Guerra, Â.F.M. (2008). Prevalence of mouth breathing among children. *Jornal de Pediatria*. **84**(5), 467–470.

Bickley, L.S. (2003). *Bates' Guide to Physical Examination and History Taking*. 8th edn. Philadelphia: Lippincott, Williams & Wilkins.

Boyton, R. & Openshaw, P. (2002). Pulmonary defences to acute respiratory infection. Oxford journals. *British Medical Bulletin*. **61**(1), 1–12.

Carden, K.A., Boiselle, P.M., Waltz, D.A. & Ernst, A. (2005). Tracheomalacia and tracheobronchomalacia in children and adults: An in-depth review. *Chest Journal*. **127**(3), 984–1005.

Clanton, T., Hogan, M. & Gladden, L. (2013). Regulation of cellular gas exchange, oxygen sensing, and metabolic control. *Comprehensive Physiology*. **3**(3), 1135–1190.

Gulati, M.S., Grewal, N. & Kaur, A. (1998). A comparative study of effects of mouth breathing and normal breathing on gingival health in children. *Journal of the Indian Society of Pedodontics and Preventive Dentistry*. **16**(3), 72–83.

Minnich, D.J. & Mathisen, D.J. (2007). Anatomy of the trachea, carina, and bronchi. *Thoracic Surgery Clinics*. **17**(4), 571–585.

Oberdörster, G. (1988). Lung clearance of inhaled insoluble and soluble particles. *Journal of Aerosol Medicine*. **1**(4), 289–330.

Pittman, R.N. (2011). *Regulation of Tissue Oxygenation*. San Rafael (CA): Morgan & Claypool Life Sciences.

Tarran, R. (2004). Regulation of airway surface liquid volume and mucus transport by active ion transport. *Proceedings of the American Thoracic Society*. **1**(1), 42–46.

Tewfik, T. & Gest, T. (2015). *Trachea Anatomy*. Medscape. http://emedicine.medscape.com/article/1949391-overview (Accessed 18.11.2016).

Tomashefsk, J. (2008). *Dail and Hammar's Pulmonary Pathology: Volume I: Nonneoplastic Lung Disease*. 3rd edn. Heidelberg: Springer Science and Business Media.

Chapter 2

Respiratory assessment

Respiratory problems are listed as one of the main reasons why patients seek medical advice and help from their doctor or nurse practitioner in primary care (British Thoracic Society 2002). Patients with undiagnosed or complicated conditions often expect a diagnosis and help with management of these conditions. To support the patient, the clinician needs to use a clinical reasoning strategy that includes a problem-solving approach in order to reach a diagnosis. One such strategy is the Barrows and Pickell model, which includes physical examination, patient involvement and education to support the clinician as they reach a diagnosis (Barrows & Pickell 1991, p. 34). The clinician collects all the information they need to make an initial concept or differential diagnosis that is accepted or rejected once they have any further information such as test results. The clinician has to be open to the idea of changing the differential diagnosis, rather than accepting it as the final answer. Diagnosis is an organic fluid process – just like the body they are assessing.

History taking

History taking is a significant part of this assessment process. It is defined as 'a conversation with a purpose' by Bickley et al. (2008). It was developed from a questioning approach to the patient's presenting complaint but has now been adapted to take a more holistic approach (Neighbour 2007, Pendleton 1993).

The primary goal of history taking is to obtain information about the patient's health and presenting problem in a structured way. This involves listening to the patient and asking appropriate questions to gain the information needed to make an informed decision about their diagnosis, their wider health and their treatment options.

The key components of history taking are: recording a patient's identifiable data, identifying their chief complaint, recording a clear timeline for their present illness, and detailing their past medical history, family history and personal and social history. It should also include a review of the other relevant systems (Bickley et al. 2008). Some would also argue that we should take time to include a spiritual history (Koenig 2004, Maugans 1996, Pulchaski & Romer 2000). It is important to take a patient's spiritual history, particularly if the patient has a life-threatening or long-term illness (Koenig, Cohen & Blazer et al. 1992).

The difference between subjective and objective data

Understanding what is subjective and what is objective information will inform your decision-making process. It will help you apply clinical reasoning to the patient scenario you are faced with. Subjective data or information is based on the patient's personal opinions, emotions and judgement. The patient may say, 'I am feeling worse'. This is considered as subjective information. Objective data or information is fact-based, which makes it more measurable and observable. An example would be recording the patient's blood pressure or pulse (Turner *et al.* 2009, p. 182).

Sometimes it can be difficult to determine whether information is subjective or objective. One method to help us take a dual approach to our history taking is to use a tool such as the MRC breathless scale (Fletcher 1952).

Table 2.1: MRC scale adapted from Fletcher (1952)

MRC Dyspnoea Scale		Your grade
Grade	**Degree of breathlessness related to activity**	
1	Not troubled by breathlessness except on strenuous exercise	
2	Short of breath when hurrying on a level or when walking up a slight hill	
3	Walks slower than most people on the level, stops after around 1.6km, or stops after 15 minutes walking at own pace	
4	Stops for breath after walking 90 metres, or after a few minutes on level ground	
5	Too breathless to leave the house, or breathless when dressing/undressing	

There are a variety of models that can be used for history taking but the components are generally the same (see Box 2.1, below).

Box 2.1: The components of history taking adapted from Bickley *et al.* (2008)

- Identifiable data
- The presenting illness
- The presenting complaint
- Past medical history
- Family history
- Personal and social history
- Spiritual history*
- Review of the other relevant systems.   *Extra topic added by author.

A history-taking method for respiratory disease

History taking involves gaining information about the whole person, to get an understanding of the patient's family and social support, their environment and their social, cultural and psychological wellbeing. At first it may appear a daunting task, but you will develop your own method of taking a history. The following method has been developed in relation to respiratory disease:

1 Identifiable data

This section speaks for itself. You need the patient's name, including the name they are usually known by. Gain their consent to the name you will identify them by. Their date of birth is also important, as this will help you determine whether the patient is a minor. Age is also important when you are considering a differential diagnosis, as some diagnoses may be age specific such as bronchiolitis.

2 Presenting illness

You may already know if the patient has a specific respiratory condition. However, it is also important to know how long they have had their illness, how the disease has progressed, and whether they have any associated conditions.

3 The presenting complaint

Although you may have identified the patient's main problem, there are two aspects to this section. You want to know the details of the presenting complaint from the patient. This should always be in the patient's own words. An example would be: 'I think I have a chest infection'. This helps you gain insight into the patient's thoughts and ideas. It makes you more aware of their perspective.

You will also want to know specific details about this complaint from a medical viewpoint. You will gain this information by specific questioning. It is important to gain a timeline for the problem. When did the patient first notice their symptoms or did someone else identify it first? For instance, they may have undiagnosed COPD, if they have had increasing breathlessness over the last year. Perhaps a partner has started to complain about a persistent night-time cough that the patient has got used to. The clinician will want to know as much as possible about this problem to make a clinical judgement about it. One method is to apply the acronym **PQRST** to the problem (Morton 1993). This stands for: **P**rovocation, **Q**uality, **R**adiates, **S**everity and **T**ime. It is often used as a tool for pain assessment but can be adapted to assess the presenting complaint (Stevens *et al.* 2011).

Provocation: What makes the problem worse or better? For instance, does the patient take an over-the-counter (OTC) cough syrup that helps their persistent cough?

Quality: Is there pain associated with the problem? Ask the patient about the extent of this pain, using a scale from 2 to 10.

Radiates: If there is pain where does it radiate to? Or are there other systems involved?

Severity: This is can be subjective. You may want to use a pain scale/tool for this. Record it in the patient's own words if possible.

Timing: When did the symptoms start? Was it a slow, gradual development or acute?

4 The past medical history

Asking about past medical history will help you put any information you gain about the patient and their condition into context. This involves asking and determining information about the patient's childhood illness, previous hospitalisation or relevant history.

5 Drug history

In this section, we want to find out what medication the patient is currently taking whether it is something they have been prescribed or they have bought over the counter.

Key questions are:

- What are you currently prescribed?
- How long have you been taking it?
- Does it make a difference to your condition?
- What medication are you allergic to?
- Do you take anything in addition to what you have been prescribed?

There are also some specific types of medication we need to be aware of. These are:

- **Non-steroidal anti-inflammatory drugs (NSAIDS):** The most common of these are aspirin, ibuprofen and naproxen and they can be prescribed or bought over the counter. Various sensitivity reactions can occur after swallowing this type of medication, ranging from IgE-mediated urticaria to angioedema and anaphylaxis. There are also a variety of non-allergic NSAID hypersensitivity syndromes which affect 0.5–1.9% of the general population. For instance, aspirin-intolerant asthma approximately affects 0.3–20% of the general population (*Allergy* 2011) and this can lead to an exacerbation of asthma and rhinitis in aspirin-induced asthma (*Allergy* 2013).

- **Beta-blockers** or **beta-adrenoceptor blocking agents**: These are medications used to control and treat conditions such as angina, atrial fibrillation, high blood pressure and heart failure. They can only be prescribed by a GP, or an independent or supplementary prescriber. In previous years, beta-blockers were considered contraindicated for patients with COPD and asthma, as there was a higher risk of bronchospasm and cough with this type of medication. Current guidance suggests that they are safe to use in this client group but that these patients need careful monitoring during their initial exposure to the drug (Morales 2014).

6 Family history

There are certainly some diseases that have a strong genetic component, such as alpha-1 antitrypsin deficiency, asthma and cystic fibrosis. Cystic fibrosis is an **autosomal recessive disease**.

In this section, we need to ask our patient a range of questions, including:

- Are the patient's parents still alive?
- If they are not alive, what was the cause of death?

- Do they have siblings? Are they well? What is their health like?

- Do the family members have a history of significant illness?

An example would be the inherited disease alpha-1 antitrypsin deficiency. If a patient has displayed the first signs of respiratory disease at a young age, and has a parent diagnosed with COPD, then one would consider alpha-1 antitrypsin deficiency as a potential differential diagnosis.

All this information can be recorded on a helpful pictorial display showing the family tree and medical history. This type of diagram is known as a genogram (see Figure 2.1).

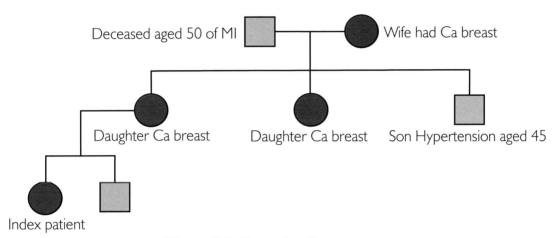

Figure 2.1: Example of a genogram

7 Psychosocial history

In this section, we also need to find out about the patient's living conditions, their occupation, their hobbies and who they live with.

- **Housing**: We want to know about their home. Do they live in a bungalow or do they need to negotiate stairs every day? Are there any environmental factors you need to be aware of, such as damp living quarters? Or do they live in the countryside, surrounded by fields of oilseed rape. All these factors help us to build a clear picture of the patient's life and identify any risks for respiratory disease.

- **Occupation**: There are a range of occupations that have an increased risk of respiratory disease associated with them (see Table 2.2 below).

- **Pets**: One also needs to know if the patient has any pets. This is significant if they have asthma or there is a question about allergic disease.

- **Hobbies**: Certain hobbies may increase the risk of developing respiratory disease, such as pigeon racing, which can lead to bird fancier's lung.

- **Lifestyle and habits**: This includes any information about smoking and intake of alcohol and non-medicinal drugs.

It is also important to assess the patient's mental state. Anxiety and depression are common in patients who have a long-term respiratory condition (Naylor *et al.* 2012). These mental health problems can certainly lead to significantly poorer health outcomes and a reduced quality of life for patients.

Table 2.2: Work-related diseases

Occupation	Associated disease and disease agent/s
Animal husbandry	Allergic asthma – straw, hay, fur
Baking	COPD – flour
Bird keeping or any association with pigeons	Bird fancier's lung – bird droppings
Building and construction	Asbestosis and mesothelioma – asbestos fibres
Coal mining	COPD and pneumoconiosis – coal dust
Diving	Small airway disease
Farming	Allergic asthma – range of triggers, from mushroom spore to wood dust Aspergillosis fungus Alveolitis – actinomycetes Farmer's lung
Paint spraying and car bodywork repairs	Asthma – isocyanates
Plastic manufacturing	Asthma – isocyanates
Quarrying industry	Silicosis – silica dust
Soldering	Asthma colophony

8 Spiritual

It is important to gain an understanding of a patient's spiritual beliefs. Religious or philosophical beliefs may affect the way a patient seeks help or interacts with those who deliver it. Their beliefs may sometimes be in conflict with their treatment plan, and this is of particular importance for end of life care. There is evidence to show that spiritual beliefs can support and help patients in the terminal stage of their disease (Spathis *et al.* 2011, p. 268).

There are tools we can use to help us make a formal spiritual assessment. One such tool is the HOPE questionnaire (Anandarajah & Hight 2001).

Box 2.2: The HOPE questionnaire

The HOPE questions for a formal spiritual assessment in a medical interview

H: What are the patient's sources of **hope**, meaning comfort, strength, peace, love and connection?

O: Are they involved in any **organised** religion?

P: What are their **personal** spiritual beliefs and practices?

E: What are the **effects** of their beliefs on medical care and end-of-life issues?

As you take a comprehensive history, you should also be observing the patient and looking for any signs or symptoms of respiratory disease. This observation will give you the clues you need to generate a hypothesis about their condition.

Box 2.3a: Reader activity

Try to identify three of the cardinal signs of respiratory disease without reading more of the text.

The three cardinal signs of respiratory disease

There are some signs and symptoms that are specifically related to the respiratory system.

I Cough: A cough is a reflex that aids the removal of foreign particles from the airway. It can be acute, or chronic (when it lasts more than 2 months). It is the most common symptom related to respiratory disease. It may have quite a trivial cause – as a post-viral cough or a symptom of **gastro-oesophageal reflux disease** (**GORD**) – or it may be an indicator of a more serious condition such as lung cancer. It is generally a reflex response to a trigger that irritates the receptors in the upper airways or larynx or trachea. It can be caused by:

- Asthma
- Bronchiectasis
- Bronchial carcinoma
- Carcinoma of the larynx and trachea
- COPD
- Cystic fibrosis
- Foreign body
- An infection, such as TB
- Post-nasal drip

- Small airways disease such as sarcoidosis, asbestosis, fibrosing alveolitis
- A viral infection, although this is usually a short-lived cough.

2 Sputum production: The amount of phlegm can increase in certain conditions, leading to the patient having to cough up sputum. The airways produce up to a teaspoon of sputum per day. A larger amount should be reviewed. Patients with the following conditions may have an increase in sputum:

- Asthma
- Bronchitis
- Bronchiectasis
- Lung cancer
- COPD
- Infection
- Sinusitis
- Smoking.

The colour and/or the odour of the sputum may also give clues to the differential diagnosis.

3 Wheeze: A wheeze is a musical sound from the airways. It is caused by the turbulence in the flow of air through the bronchi and bronchioles. It can be related to inspiration or expiration. It is a common symptom in obstructive respiratory disease such as asthma.

Thick white sputum indicates inflammation of the airway, whereas suppurative green sputum would indicate a significant infection. If the patient coughs up blood, this is considered a medical emergency or 'a red flag'.

Haemoptysis

When a patient coughs up blood, one has to consider that there may be significant pathology. Fresh blood may come from the oral cavity but if it is mixed with sputum it is more likely to be coming from the upper airways. The most common causes in adults are lung cancer, tuberculosis or pneumonia; children are more likely to cough up blood due to the inhalation of a foreign body in the airway.

Table 2.2: Causes of cough

Type of cough	Diagnostic indicator
Bubbly or frothy	Left-hearted heart failure (LHF)
Dry cough	Allergic rhinitis and post-nasal drip
Dry hacking cough	Mycoplasma pneumonia

Productive cough	Upper respiratory infection Lower respiratory infection Bronchitis Pneumonia Bacterial or viral infection
Distinctive coughs (e.g. whooping cough)	**Pertussis** (whooping cough)
Night-time cough	LHF and asthma

Types of breathlessness

Breathlessness is a distressing and uncomfortable symptom, due to a deficit between the body's demand for air and the ability of the respiratory system to satisfy that demand. It is classified as:

A: Acute breathlessness, which can develop over a few minutes, hours or days (< 2 weeks)

B: Chronic breathlessness, which can develop over several weeks or months? (> 3 months).

Breathlessness that develops within minutes may be due to:

- Acute asthma
- Cardiac rhythm problem
- Dissecting aneurysm
- **Pneumothorax**
- Pulmonary emboli.

Breathlessness that develops over hours or days may be due to:

- Asthma
- Cardiac valve disorder
- Haemorrhage
- Left ventricular failure (LVF)
- **Pleural effusion**.

Breathlessness that develops over weeks or months may be due to:

- **Anaemia**
- Fibrosing alveolitis
- Malignancy
- Obesity
- Respiratory muscle weakness
- Valve dysfunction.

It is therefore important to identify the underlying cause of breathlessness. Determining whether it is acute or chronic will also affect your decision. You may want more information from additional tests and assessments. A chest x-ray may help you identify signs of heart failure and pleural effusion. An electrocardiogram (ECG) will help you determine whether there are signs of heart failure, arrhythmia, and pulmonary embolism. Other tests are a full blood count to check for anaemia and C-reactive protein or erythrocyte sedimentation rate (ESR) to check for evidence of infection (NICE 2010).

Box 2.4a: Reader activity

List five causes of acute breathlessness.

This framework should give you the information you need. It is also important to use key verbal and non-verbal communication skills. One example would be to use open-ended questions so the patient can explain in their own words, rather than closed questions eliciting a simple yes or no. The consultation can also be viewed as a therapeutic relationship so it is important to be empathetic and supportive (Bickley *et al.* 2008, p. 75). This may give you an insight into some of your patient's real concerns about their health and wellbeing.

Having used this structured approach to history taking, you can start to draw up a list of potential differential diagnoses, which can be reviewed during the next stage of assessment.

Summary

Following a brief explanation of objective and subjective data, this chapter has introduced an eight-stage model of history taking which can be adapted in particular practice situations. The information gained during this process should help you formulate a list of potential diagnoses.

Table 2.4: Specific areas to consider, relating to respiratory disease

Areas to be addressed	
Smoking habits	Record smoking of cigarettes, cigars or pipe. Age when patient started to smoke, number of cigarettes smoked per day and estimate of total 'pack-years'* of smoking.
Current smoking status	If patient is an ex-smoker, include date when patient stopped smoking. If not, was there any attempt to discontinue smoking in the past? Also include details of any illicit substances that are smoked.
Environmental review	Carry out a chronological review of occupational exposure to triggers, including specific environmental and work exposure.
Cough	Is the cough intermittent or every day (seldom or only nocturnal)? A night-time cough may indicate LHF or asthma.
Nature of cough	Is the cough productive or non-productive (especially on awakening)? How much sputum is the patient producing? Are they coughing up blood? Frank or old? Are there streaks of blood?
Chest pain	Localise the pain. Does it radiate elsewhere? Describe the onset. How long does it last for? Is the pain progressive?
Sputum production	Document the amount of sputum produced per day. Is it a teaspoon or more? Is there a foul taste? This could indicate the presence of infection.
Dyspnoea	Progressive and present every day? Use tool.
Presence of laboured breathing	Is this exercise related? Does it result in progressive limitation of activity? Is the patient's breathing laboured even at rest?
Precipitants other than exercise, especially respiratory infection	
Wheezing	Frequency and duration, diurnal pattern, factors precipitating the problem. This may include weather, house dust, etc.
Acute respiratory infections	What is the frequency and timing of acute infections? Check for the presence of cough, dyspnoea, sputum and sputum purulence, wheezing and fever.
Requiring treatment such as antibiotics or systemic corticosteroids	

*The number of pack-years can be calculated as: Number of pack-years = number of packs of cigarettes per day, multiplied by number of years of smoking (e.g. one pack of 20 cigarettes).

Box 2.3b: Answers to reader activity

The three cardinal signs of respiratory disease are:

1. Cough

2. Sputum production

3. Wheeze.

Box 2.4b: Answers to reader activity

Causes of acute breathlessness can include:

- Acute asthma
- Acute exacerbation of COPD
- Airway obstruction
- Bronchiectasis
- Community-acquired pneumonia
- Diabetic ketoacidosis
- Lung/lobar collapse
- Pleural effusion
- Psychogenic breathlessness
- Pulmonary embolism
- Trauma
- Thyroxicosis.

References

Anandarajah, G. & Hight, E. (2001). Spirituality and medical practice: Using the HOPE questions as a practical tool for spiritual assessment. *American Family Physician*. **63**(1), 81–89.

Allergy. (July 2011) 66(7), 818–29. doi: 10.1111/j.1398-9995.2011.02557

Allergy. (October 2013) 68(10), 1219–1232. doi: 10.1111/all.12260

Barrows, H. & Pickell, G. (1991). *Developing clinical problem solving skills: A guide to more effective diagnosis and treatment*. New York: Norton Medical Books.

Bickley, L.S., Szilagyi, P.G. & Bates, B. (2008). *Bates' guide to physical examination and history taking*. Philadelphia: USA. Lippincott, Williams & Wilkins.

British Thoracic Society (BTS) (2002). The burden of disease. *Epidemiology*. **107**, 357.

Fletcher, C.M. (1952). The clinical diagnosis of pulmonary emphysema—an experimental study. *Proceedings of the Royal Society of Medicine*. **45**, 577–584.

Koenig, H.G. (2004). Taking a spiritual history. *Journal of the American Medical Association*. **291**(23), 2881–2882.

Koenig, H.G., Cohen, H.J., Blazer, D.G. *et al.* (1992). Religious coping and depression among elderly, hospitalized medically ill men. *American Journal of Psychiatry*. **149**, 693–1700.

Maugans, T.A. (1996). The spiritual history. *Archives of Family Medicine*. **5**(1), 11–16.

Morales, D. (2014). Initiating beta-blockers in patients with asthma. *Prescriber*. http://onlinelibrary.wiley.com/doi/10.1002/psb.1249/pdf (Accessed 23.11.2016).

Naylor, C., Parsonage, M., McDaid, D., Knapp, M., Fossey, M. & Galea, A. (2012). *Long-term conditions and mental health. The cost of co-morbidities*. The King's Fund. http://www.kingsfund.org.uk/sites/files/kf/field/field_publication_file/long-term-conditions-mental-health-cost-comorbidities-naylor-feb12.pdf (Accessed 23.11.2016).

Neighbour, R. (2007). *The Inner Consultation: How to Develop an Effective and Intuitive Consulting Style*. Oxford: Radcliffe.

NICE (2010). *Breathlessness; NICE Clinical Knowledge Summaries*. http://cks.nice.org.uk/breathlessness (Accessed 23.11.2016).

Pendleton, D., Schofield, T., Tate. P. & Havelock, P. (2003). *The New Consultation: Developing Doctor Patient Communication*. Oxford: Oxford University Press.

Primary Care Respiratory Society (PCRS) (2015). *The dyspnoea scale*. https://www.pcrs-uk.org/mrc-dyspnoea-scale (Accessed 23.11.2016).

Puchalski, C. & Romer, A.L. (2000). Taking a spiritual history allows clinicians to understand patients more fully. *Journal of Palliative Medicine*. **3**(1), 129–137.

Spathis, A., Booth, S. & Davies, H.E. (2011). *Respiratory Disease: From Advanced Disease to Bereavement*. Oxford: Oxford University Press.

Stevens, B., Abbott, L. K., Yamada, J., Harrison, D., Stinson, J., Taddio, A., Finley, G.A. for the CIHR Team in Children's Pain. (2011). Epidemiology and management of painful procedures in children in Canadian Hospitals. *Canadian Medical Association Journal*. **183**(7), E403–E410.

Chapter 3

Physical assessment

This chapter reviews the physical assessment skills you need to use when assessing a patient with respiratory disease. The process starts, like any initial encounter, when you first see or hear the patient. We often make assumptions and assess someone without even realising it. For instance, you may hear the patient wheezing or coughing as they walk down a corridor towards you. You can therefore be intentional about your assessment during this period.

The physical examination should start with a general examination of the patient. This means that you do not focus only on the system the patient is complaining about. As with any physical examination, the clinician needs to use a structured approach. The order of assessment is:

● Inspection
● Palpation
● Percussion
● Auscultation.

The patient should be informed about what you will be doing. They should be made to feel relaxed and in control. The patient will need to be undressed for you to do a thorough assessment. You cannot observe chest wall movement, for example, if they have a vest on. It is also helpful to be mindful of the basic anatomical landmarks of the chest when you are preparing to perform a physical examination, with particular focus on the respiratory system.

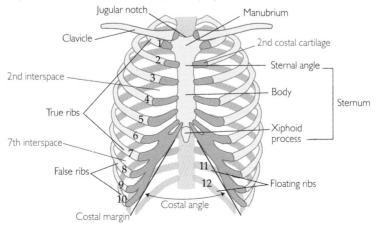

Figure 3.1: The anatomical landmarks of the chest

Vital signs

- **Pulse**: A bounding pulse is a sign of CO_2 retention.
- **Respiratory rate**: The respiratory rate for a healthy adult is 10–14 breaths per minute. An increase in this rate can be found in a number of disorders, ranging from anxiety to pneumonia and heart failure. This is an important clinical observation, as a rise in a patient's respiratory rate can be an indicator of their deterioration. It is also a sensitive observation. **Tachypnoea** is the term used for an increase in respiratory rate above the norm. It indicates that the body has identified an increase in its oxygen requirement. This can be due to illness or if someone undertakes exercise.
- **Respiratory pattern**: The normal pattern of breathing is regulated on an unconscious level. A rapid and deep pattern can be an indicator of metabolic **acidosis**. **Cheyne Stokes breathing** involves deeper depths of inspiration or expiration. This can occur with patients who have cerebral or respiratory depression or cardiac failure or who are at the end of life.

General inspection

This is a systematic general assessment of the patient that should start the moment you see them. It should only take a few minutes. From this you can ascertain a rough age, the patient's general health, the environment they are in and whether they are acutely ill or not. Inspection is therefore the first and most important aspect in a physical examination.

Skin

- In the early stages of sarcoidosis and also in primary tuberculosis, patients can present with **erythema nodosum** on the skin. In this condition, inflamed fat cells lead to painful, reddish, tender lumps, mainly on the shins. The nodules can vary in size from 1 to 5 centimetres.
- Does the patient appear to have muscle wasting or a reduced **body mass index (BMI)**?
- Do they have **atopic eczema**? This is often found on the face and limbs.

Hands

When assessing the hands, look for the following signs and symptoms:

- **Cyanosis** is the name given to the bluish tinge on the extremities, when there is a reduction in oxygenated **haemoglobin (Hb)** in the circulating blood cells.
- **Finger clubbing** is an important clinical sign that can occur with a significant number of chronic respiratory disorders. The tissue at the base of the nail thickens and obliterates the angle between the nail bed and the adjacent skin of the finger. It can occur due to pulmonary, cardiac, hepatic or gastrointestinal causes.
- **Asterixis** is finger flapping (also known as the flapping tremor) and is a tremor of the hand

when the wrist is extended. Asterixis is due to **encephalopathies** and faulty metabolism. It is also a sign of CO_2 retention.

- There may be nicotine staining of the nails and fingers. You may also notice peripheral cyanosis, where there is a bluish colour to the skin and mucous membranes, due to low levels of circulating O_2.

Face

- Eyes will indicate whether or not the patient has **Horner's syndrome**. The pupil constricts and there is **ptosis** (muscle weakness), increased sweating and inset eyeball, as a result of carcinoma of the **bronchi**.
- The mucous membranes in the mouth and tongue may be cyanosed. You should also check the underside of the tongue for any colour change.
- Pallor of the **conjunctivae** can indicate **anaemia**.

Chest and neck.

- The patient may be in some degree of respiratory distress and may have to use their **accessory muscles**.
- Assess **jugular venous pressure** (**JVP**). Ask the patient to sit with their torso at a 45-degree angle (semi-recumbent). The patient should have their head and neck resting on a pillow. Get them to turn their head to face left. You are looking for the pulsation of the right jugular vein. The landmarks are the internal jugular vein, which runs from the medial end of the **clavicle** to the ear lobe. You may see a double pulsation. You can assess the JVP by measuring the vertical distance between the sternal angle and the JVP, which should be less than 3cm.
- Assess the cervical lymph nodes. Palpate the areas to assess if they are enlarged, which is a sign of infection or illness.
- The **trachea** should be centrally placed. If it is displaced, this is a sign of pulmonary collapse. You can also ask the patient to take a deep breath; if the trachea moves downwards during inspiration, this can be a sign of severe **chronic obstructive pulmonary disorder** (**COPD**), also called a **tracheal tug**.
- Assess the chest shape.
  - **Scoliosis** this is a condition that causes the spine to curve to the left or right sides. It usually develops during puberty.
  - **Kyphosis** is a condition where there is excessive convex curvature of the spine.
  - **Barrel chest** is a term used to describe a rounded, bulging chest that reminds us of the shape of a barrel.
  - **Pectus carinatum**

- **Pectus excavatum**
- **Harrison's sulcus.**

Breathing patterns

Listen to the patient as you introduce yourself. They may have difficulty in breathing, in which case they will be using their accessory muscles, or you can hear them wheezing. Assess whether the wheeze occurs during inspiration or expiration. Consider the breathing pattern. Do they have **Kussmaul breathing** when you hear them deeply sighing? They may have Cheyne Stokes respiration, which is alternate rapid breaths and shallow ones. This pattern is often heard at the end of life or if a patient is acutely ill. If the patient has a partial obstruction, you may hear a harsh vibrating noise when they breathe called **stridor**. This is a medical emergency.

Palpation

You can assess chest expansion by placing your hands on the patient's upper chest. Your thumbs should sit in line with the **axillae** and the thumbs parallel to each other. As the patient breathes in and out, so the distance increases or decreases between the thumbs. This simple action is a helpful indicator of chest symmetry and it can be repeated on the patient's back.

Tactile fremitus

The normal **lung** tissue can transmit a vibratory sensation to the chest wall and this is called **fremitus**. To assess this, the clinician can place the ulnar side of their hands firmly on both sides of the chest. During tactile fremitus, we ask the patient to repeat the words 'ninety- nine'. If the lung tissue is filled with fluid or air, the fremitus becomes more pronounced. A fluid-filled space, such as a **pleural effusion**, can decrease fremitus.

Once you have completed the palpation, you can progress to percussion.

Percussion

Percussion is used to determine what is underneath the surface. To perform this technique, you need to use the middle finger, or the middle finger and adjoining finger of one hand, tapping on the middle finger of the other, flicking the wrist as you do it. The non-striking finger is placed over the area you are assessing.

When percussing the patient's chest, work your way across from side to side, comparing right to left. You can practise your technique by percussing a solid object and a hollow object. Listen to the sounds. A solid object will sound dull. There are four types of percussion sounds (Thomas & Monaghan 2007, p. 214):

- Resonant – normal lung sound
- Hyper-resonant – this is the sound made by an area of reduced density, such as an air-filled structure

- Stony dull – this is an extreme dull sound, perhaps found over a pleural effusion
- Dull – this sound is due to the presence of a solid mass or bone.

Start the percussion phase of chest examination by tapping over the clavicle bones on each side (these are the apices of the lung). Then move downwards from side to side, listening to each sound. Repeat on the front and the back of the chest. Look for symmetry and any unexpected notes.

Auscultation

Before you listen to the chest, it is helpful to know where to place your stethoscope and what type of sounds you are listening for. The stethoscope amplifies the sounds that originate within the chest. The bell of the stethoscope is used to hear low-frequency sounds and is ideal to use for small children or thin people. The diaphragm is best used for high-frequency sounds. Start with the anterior chest wall.

The bell part of the stethoscope should be placed above the apices of the lungs, in the supraclavicular area. Ask the patient to take deep breaths in out of their mouth. Listen to the sound through the stethoscope on one side, then the other. Swap to the diaphragm over the remaining areas.

The minimum number of places to listen would be in four areas on either side of the chest (i.e. a total of eight). As you are undertaking this procedure, consider where you are placing your stethoscope and consider what lobe of the lung is where. Once you have listened to the back of the chest, move to the front, repeating the process. You should also ask the patient to take some slow deep breaths, as you are listening for the breathing sounds.

A healthy person will produce soft inspiratory sounds as the air enters the airways. There is less sound made on expiration. This is called **vesicular breathing**. See the following table for further breath sounds you may hear.

Table 3.1: Breathe sounds

Breath sounds	Presentation	Example of condition
Bronchial	These are laryngeal sounds, which are transmitted to the chest wall if there is solid matter present.	Consolidation, as in infection **Fibrosis** Airway collapse, as in **pneumothorax**
Diminished volume	Reduced transmission of sound.	**Atelectasis** COPD Obesity Pleural effusion (sounds may be absent over this) Pleural thickening
Vesicular	The breath sounds get louder during inspiration, and fade with expiration.	Normal breathing pattern

Table 3.2: Adventitious abnormal sounds

Additional sounds	Notes	Condition
Crepitation	Heard during inspiration. Can be heard in early or late inspiration.	Pneumonia
Rhonchi (wheezing)		Asthma
Pleural rub		Pleurisy
Egophony (vocal resonance)		There is increased vocal resonance with lung consolidation or fibrosis.
Whispering pectoriloquy	See assessment tests.	Loud transmission is heard above the level of fluid in patients with a pleural effusion.

Vocal resonance

Vocal resonance is also known as pectoriloquy and is similar to vocal fremitus, (Epstein *et al.* 2004). The aim of this procedure is to listen to the transmission of the sound from the lungs. Ask the patient to say 'ninety-nine', which is the English translation from the German physician who first devised the test. Then listen to the patient as they say this with the stethoscope in the upper, mid and lower zones of the chest. Increased resonance is due to the presence of fluid in the alveolar spaces. A decrease in resonance can be caused by fluid or air in the pleural sac – **pneumothorax**. The sound is therefore muffled. The patient is then asked to repeat the test but this time they are asked to whisper the words 'ninety-nine'.

Once the examination is completed and the findings are recorded, the clinician can make a list of differential diagnoses. There may only be one provisional diagnosis. The next step is to determine what other information or clues you need to reach a final diagnosis. To do this, you may need further secondary data. However, if there is a clear diagnosis, a treatment plan can be devised – in partnership with the patient and/or their family.

Summary

In this chapter, we have discussed the structured approach to chest examination. We have looked at inspection, palpation, percussion and auscultation of the chest and reviewed the normal and potential abnormal findings. This is summarised in the following table. However, chest examination is only part of the process of determining the patient's diagnosis.

Table 3.3: Respiratory chest examination checklist

		Findings
1	Introduces self.	
2	Adopts client-centred approach.	
3	Gains consent for removal of shirt.	
4	Inspects for signs of anaemia.	
5	Inspects for signs of cyanosis.	
6	Checks respiratory rate.	
7	Checks position of trachea.	
8	Checks for use of respiratory muscles.	
9.	Checks for spinal deformities, scars, etc.	
10.	Checks hands for finger clubbing.	
11.	Listens for wheeze.	
12.	Inspects anterior and posterior chest.	
13.	Demonstrates appropriate technique for palpation.	
14.	Assesses the expansion and symmetry of the chest.	
15.	Checks for tactile fremitus, both anterior and posterior.	
16.	Demonstrates appropriate percussion technique, both anterior and posterior.	
17.	States sound heard over normal tissue.	
18.	States sound heard over bone.	
19.	States sound heard over solid mass.	
20.	Demonstrates appropriate auscultation technique.	
21.	States listening for adventitious sounds – crackles.	
22.	States listening for adventitious sounds – ronchi (wheezing).	
23.	States listening for adventitious sounds – pleural rub.	
24.	Demonstrates or describes (bronchiloquy) Bronchophony which is a form of pectoriloquy.	
25.	Demonstrates or describes whispered pectoriloquy.	
26.	Demonstrates or describes egophony.	

References

Epstein, O., Perkin, G., Cookson, J. & de Bono, D. (2004). *Pocket Guide to Clinical Examination.* 3rd edn. Mosby: Edinburgh.

Thomas, J. & Monaghan, T. (2007). *Oxford Handbook of Clinical Examination and Practical Skills.* Oxford: Oxford University Press.

Turner, R., Angus, B., Handa, A. & Hatton, C. (2009). *Clinical Skills and Examination.* Oxford: Wiley-Blackwell.

Chapter 4

Secondary data

Secondary data is needed in the diagnostic and assessment process to validate patient symptoms and aid the clinician in the problem-solving process. The data can be obtained through specific tests, indices and observations. These test results help us in the process of supporting or rejecting the hypothesis generated during the assessment process.

This can be seen in the following case study.

A 66-year-old retired teacher attended the surgery complaining of increased shortness of breath (SOB) over the past six months. She had a history of winter bronchitis. There was no other significant history apart from mild hay fever in the summer months. No family history and no social history concerns. She was a non-smoker, although her parents had been heavy smokers. Her peak flows were below expected. There was an audible wheeze on chest examination but no other symptoms. Her diagnosis was possible chronic obstructive pulmonary disorder (COPD) or undiagnosed asthma. Further data was needed to confirm or reject the diagnosis.

Secondary data was obtained from her spirometry results, which showed a restrictive pattern. After further x-ray and computed tomography (CT) scanning, it was found she had lymphoma.

The following table lists a number of respiratory conditions and some of the tests used to identify them.

Table 4.1: Specific tests

Disease	Investigations
Asthma	Spirometry with reversibility Blood tests – total and specific **immunoglobulin E** Skin testing with **allergens** **Radioallergosorbent (RAST) testing**
Cystic fibrosis	Sweat tests Gene studies

Extrinsic allergic alveolitis	Blood test for specific precipitating **antibodies**
Emphysema (inherited)	Blood test: **alpha 1-antitrypsin**
Pleural effusion	Chest x-ray Total protein, **lactate dehydrogenase (LDH)**, glucose, cholesterol and others in pleural fluid
Pneumonia	Chest x-ray **C-reactive protein (CRP) + erythrocyte sedimentation rate (ESR)** **Sputum** microscopy CRB65/CURB65 score
Pulmonary embolism	Blood tests: clotting factors, D-dimer and imaging **Antineutrophil cytoplasmic antibodies (ANCA)**
(Latent) tuberculosis infection	Tuberculin skin test, interferon-gamma release assays
Lung cancer	Chest x-ray CT scan Tumour markers – CEA, CYFRA 21-1, NSE, SCC **Positron emission tomography (PET) scan**
Malignant mesothelioma	Chest x-ray Tumour markers
Sarcoidosis	**Angiotensin-converting enzyme (ACE)**
Unexplained breathlessness	Haemoglobin **N-terminal pro b-type natriuretic peptide (NT-proBNP)** – increase in heart failure

Blood tests

Blood test results are helpful to the clinician, as they are used to confirm or reject the diagnosed cause of disease or they are related to the symptoms a patient is experiencing.

Alpha-1 antitrypsin

One specific respiratory blood test is for alpha-1 antitrypsin (AIAT) deficiency. Alpha-1 antitrypsin (AIAT) deficiency is one of the most common inherited disorders among white people and is thought to be the causative factor in 1–3% of cases of COPD (Dirksen 1999). It also has a high prevalence in Northwest Europe (Coakley *et al.* 2001). In the UK, it is estimated that 1:5,000 people have AIAT deficiency. **It is thought to be the causative factor in 1–3% of people diagnosed with COPD** (Fairman *et al.* 2011).

It is helpful to investigate the serum levels of AIAT in order to reach a diagnosis. The serum levels are usually between 20 and 60 mmol/L but if the level falls below 11μmol/L then the disorder can cause tissue damage. **Phenotyping** should be carried out on those with low serum levels. Liver function tests should also be considered.

Haematocrit

The **haematocrit** level tells the clinician what the **packed cell volume** (**PCV**) is, as a percentage of the circulating red blood cells. In men, this should be 45% and women slightly lower at 40% (Purves *et al.* 2004, p. 954). This is a helpful investigation for **polycythaemia**, which causes an increase in red blood cells. Secondary polycythaemia is a recognised condition that can occur with patients with COPD and can lead to **pulmonary hypertension**. It is also a risk factor for stroke (Kent *et al.* 2011). Treatment may include the removal of blood from the circulation.

Full blood count

The **full blood count** (**FBC**) measures the amount of haemoglobin and the haematocrit levels and specific white cells (see Table 4.2). White blood cells are an indicator of the presence of inflammation and/or infection. Haemoglobin is the iron-rich protein in red blood cells that carries oxygen and a low level of it may indicate that the patient is anaemic. It is a helpful test when you want to rule out other causes of breathlessness.

- The normal haemoglobin level for men is: 13.8−17.2g/dL
- The normal haemoglobin level for women is: 12.1−15.1g/dL

The FBC also looks at a patient's **mean corpuscular volume** (MCV). This is a measure of the average size of the patient's red blood cells and is a helpful test for the cause of **anaemia**. In iron deficiency anaemia, red blood cells can be smaller in size than normal so clients can have a low MCV.

- The normal MCV is: 80−100fL.

Table 4.2: Full blood count results

Blood test		Normal reference range	Units of measurement
Haemoglobin	Adult male Adult female	130−180 115−165	g/L g/L
Total white cell count	Adult	3.6−11.0	x10^9/L
Neutrophils **Lymphocytes** **Monocytes** **Eosinophils** **Basophils**	Adult Adult Adult Adult Adult	1.8−7.5 1.0−4.0 0.2−0.8 0.1−0.4 0.02−0.1	x10^9/L
Platelet count	Adult	140−400	x10^9/L
Red cell count	Male Female	4.50−6.50 3.80−5.80	x10^{12}/L x10^{12}/L
Haematocrit	Male Female	0.40−0.54 0.37−0.47	L/L L/L
Mean corpuscular volume (MCV)	Adult	80−100	fL
Mean cell haemoglobin (MCH)	Adult	27−32	Pg

Blood gas analysis

An **arterial blood gas** (**ABG**) analysis measures the arterial oxygen tension (PaO_2) and ($PaCO_2$). It also gives the clinician information on the **acid-base balance** at a specific point in a patient's illness. The blood is taken directly from the **radial artery**, as the superficial anatomic presentation of this vessel makes it easily accessible.

An ABG analysis is generally carried out:

- To assess for severe asthma, cystic fibrosis, or COPD). Patients with a **forced expiratory volume in one second** (**FEV1**) < 40% of predicted require an ABG; likewise patients whose SaO_2 is < 92% on two or more occasions.
- To assess oxygen requirement for those receiving O_2 therapy.
- To measure the acid-base status of people who have heart failure, kidney failure, uncontrolled diabetes or patients on an insulin pump, or suffering from sleep disorders or severe infections, or after a drug overdose.
- To assess patients who are receiving therapeutic treatment such as ventilation.

Usual results

The partial pressure of oxygen (PaO_2) in arterial blood is usually > 11kPa.

The partial pressure of carbon dioxide ($PaCO_2$) in arterial blood is usually between 4.7 and 6kPa.

The pH of the blood is in the normal range (7.35–7.45).

You need to know how to interpret blood gases and remember that acidosis or alkalosis may be present, even if the pH is in the normal range (Kaufman 2015).

Sputum cultures

Sputum is the name given to the **mucus** and other phlegm that is coughed up from the airways. It is a helpful indicator as to the presence of infection or other causes of disease. The best time to collect a sputum sample is in the morning, as the sample is likely to be more concentrated. It is important to note the colour, consistency and odour of the sample.

The types of sputum you may see are:

- Purulent sputum, which is typically yellow or green in colour. It contains white blood cells, cellular debris, serous fluid and mucus. It is typically seen when patients have **bronchiectasis**, bronchitis or acute upper respiratory tract infection. A yellow-greenish colour suggests that treatment with antibiotics can reduce symptoms, as the green colour is caused by degenerating neutrophil Myeloperoxidase.
- Bloody sputum or **haemoptysis**, which can take one of three forms:
  - Blood-streaked sputum or haemoptysis – can be due to inflammation of throat or **bronchi** caused by infection, trauma or lung cancer

- Pink sputum – sputum mixed with blood from the small or peripheral airways
- A large amount of blood – due to tuberculosis, lung cancer, severe infection or pulmonary embolism.
- Rust coloured – usually caused by pneumonia, pulmonary embolism, lung cancer or pulmonary tuberculosis.
- Brown – caused by chronic bronchitis (greenish/yellowish/brown), chronic pneumonia (whitish-brown), tuberculosis or lung cancer.
- White/grey sputum colour – due to an acute inflammatory infection such as allergic bronchitis.
- Opaque, mucoid or white – an indicator of a viral infection.
- Foamy white – earlier phase pulmonary oedema.
- Frothy pink – severe pulmonary oedema.

Currently, routine testing of sputum culture for patients with chronic respiratory disease is only recommended if they are admitted to hospital and when the sputum is purulent (NICE). This is because a percentage of patients with a stable respiratory disease, as in COPD, have chronic colonisation of their airways (Monso et al. 1995, Stockley et al. 2000). A more accurate test would be **bronchoscopic alveolar lavage** (**BAL**) and microscopy.

Chest x-rays

Radiography involves making film records (radiographs) of the body's internal structures. There are several different types of radiography, including tomography, electron radiography and neutron radiography which produce two dimensional medical images (Turner et al. 2009). The images can be read and interpreted and stored for future reference. Chest radiography can be challenging, as there are so many potentially visible pathologies. These x-rays are therefore generally not routinely recommended.

However, they are requested for:

- Suspected pneumomediastinium or **pneumothorax**
- Suspected consolidation
- Patients with life-threatening asthma
- Patients who fail to respond to treatment satisfactorily
- Patients who require ventilation.

The x-ray should be taken in the posterior–anterior position, as this helps to give an accurate picture of the heart edges (Turner et al. 2009, p. 203). The x-ray should be taken during inspiration when the six anterior ribs are above the diaphragm. The thoracic spine should be in the centre of the **sternum** and between the **clavicles**. The outlines should be sharp. The outline of the **mediastinum** should be smooth. It should also be centrally located in the chest. One would expect the lungs to be of equal density. The **hilar** (or lung roots) consist of the major bronchi, pulmonary veins and arteries, which should be visible. The hilar lymph nodes are not usually visible on x-ray. One should also be able to assess the size and shape of the aorta, nodes and any enlarged vessels. The heart will be visible, right of the midline. If the thoracic diameter is over half of the thoracic width this is an indication of an enlarged heart. Particular care should be taken to identify the lung apices.

When looking at x-rays of the lungs, one has to consider:

- Size
- Shape
- Silhouette
- Diameter.

Indicators of abnormality:

- Infiltrates
- Increased interstitial markings
- Masses
- Absence of normal margins
- **Bronchograms**
- Increased vascularity.

Lung function tests

There is a wide range of lung function tests. Assessing a patient's **peak expiratory rate (peak flow)** is the most common of these tests and one that you do not need to have additional training for (GOLD 2015). It simply records how fast an individual can breathe out.

The peak flow is measured using a standardised EU peak flow meter. The patient is asked to stand up and hold the meter, taking care not to place their fingers over the dial. They are then asked to take a deep breath in, seal their mouth around the disposable mouthpiece and exhale sharply. The dial will record their peak expiratory rate in litres per minute. The aim is to obtain three similar readings and to record the best of the three.

Spirometry is a specific test to assess lung function. It is recommended that you use post-bronchodilator spirometry to diagnose the presence of irreversible or limited airflow obstruction (GOLD 2015).

This can be a difficult and trying test to perform so there are some exclusion criteria for those who perform it. The patient can potentially be harmed, due to the pressures generated in the thorax and their impact on the abdominal and thoracic organs. There can also be significant changes in blood pressure, causing stresses on vital organs. There are also potential concerns regarding the expansion of the chest wall and lungs, as in the case of a patient who has had recent abdominal surgery. Spirometry should *not* be performed if a patient has a communicable disease such as tuberculosis (Cooper 2010). The test should of course be carried out by someone who has been taught how to do the test and interpret the results (GOLD 2015).

The following results are recorded during spirometry testing:

- The **forced vital capacity** (**FVC**) is the volume of air that is breathed out following maximal inspiration. This should be performed within 3 seconds and 75% of this volume should be blown out in the first second. If a patient has an obstructive disease, they can breathe out the volume but it will take longer to do so. The FVC is the total volume of air that the patient can forcibly exhale in one breath.

- The volume breathed out in the first second is called the forced expiratory volume in one second (FEVI). The FEVI/FVC ratio is a calculated ratio and it represents the proportion of a person's vital capacity that they are able to expire in the first second of forced expiration.

The FEVI and FVC are also expressed as a percentage of the predicted normal exhalation for a person of the same sex, age and height (British Thoracic Society 2005). An FEVI/FVC of < 70% indicates obstructive disease (NICE 2010).

Table 4.3: Severity of airflow obstruction

Severity of airflow obstruction (Stage)	Stage 1: Mild	Stage 2: Moderate	Stage 3: Severe	Stage 4: Very severe
FEVI (% predicted)	≥ 80 + symptoms	50–79	39–49	< 50 + respiratory failure or < 30

Gas transfer testing

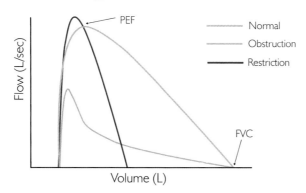

Figure 4.1: Flow graphs

You can also assess the transfer of gases from the lungs to the bloodstream by using a marker gas that can be traced. T_LCO testing is certainly something that should be considered if symptoms in COPD are disproportionate to the spirometric values and for other obstructive diseases (GOLD 2015, Mims 2010). The test may help characterise the severity of COPD but can also be used as an adjunct to other tests. This is a non-invasive test. The patient simply has to breathe in, using a mouthpiece connected to a spirometer and gas containers. They have to rapidly inhale (to vital capacity inspiration) a set mixture of gases that contain 0.3% CO, 14% helium (He) and 18% O_2. The patient is asked to hold their breath for 10 seconds and then asked to perform a rapid expiration. A set amount of the expired gas is then analysed for CO and helium.

Allergen testing

One of the most common tests used for allergy asthma is the skin prick test. This looks for specific antigen responses and sensitivity to common allergens.

The patient has their forearm cleaned with alcohol. The arm is then labelled with the name of each allergen on one side and a histamine-based control on the opposite side. There is a wide range of antigens that can be used, from grass pollen and cat dander to nuts. The patient must not take any antihistamine medication for at least 48 hours prior to the test. They then receive a miniscule amount of allergen in an aqueous solution. A fine lancet is used to pierce the skin, through the allergen solution, and the excess solution is removed. The patient then has to sit and wait for 15 minutes. If there is a reaction, the patient develops a wheal 2mm larger than the control. Although this form of testing is commonly used, RAST testing (using blood samples) is becoming more popular because it is so easy to carry out.

Exercise testing

Exercise testing can be objectively carried out by assessing the reduction in a self-paced walking distance or during an incremental exercise programme in a Physiology Laboratory (Carter et al. 2003, Pinto-Plata et al. 2004). The 2-Minute Walk Test (2MWT) has been shown to be reliable when assessing exercise capacity in patients with respiratory disease (Leung et al. 2006). It can also be used to determine the deterioration of lung function and as an indicator of mortality (Carter et al. 2003, Pinto-Plata et al. 2004) because exercise capacity has been shown to fall the year prior to death (Polkey et al. 2013).

Composite methods

Measuring exercise capacity can also form part of a composite scoring system or tool such as BODE (standing for BMI, obstruction, dyspnoea and exercise). This method gives a composite score for a patient's body mass index, obstruction (forced expiratory volume in 1 second), dyspnoea and exercise (Celli et al. 2004). See Box 4.1 (the BODE method) and Box 4.2 (the approximate 4-year survival interpretation).

Summary

There are many tests you can use to help diagnose and manage patients with respiratory illness. Some of these tests are more reliable, and can be clearly interpreted more easily, than others. However, all test results need to be reviewed in the light of the whole assessment process and your knowledge of the patient as an individual.

Box 4.1: The BODE method

Select criteria:
FEV1 % Predicted after bronchodilator

- $> = 65\%$ (0 points)
- 50–64% (1 point)
- 36–49% (2 points)
- $< = 35\%$ (3 points)

6-minute walk distance

- $> = 350$ metres (0 points)
- 250–349 metres (1 point)
- 150–249 metres (2 points)
- $< = 149$ metres (3 points)

MMRC dyspnoea scale (4 is worst)

- MMRC 0: Dyspnoeic on strenuous exercise (0 points)
- MMRC 1: Dyspnoeic on walking a slight hill (0 points)
- MMRC 2: Dyspnoeic on walking on level ground; must stop occasionally due to breathlessness (1 point)
- MMRC 3: Must stop for breathlessness after walking 90 metres (100 yards) or after a few minutes (2 points)
- MMRC 4: Cannot leave house; breathless on dressing/undressing (3 points)

Body mass index

- > 21 (0 points)
- $< = 21$ (1 point)

Results: Total criteria point count:

Box 4.2: The approximate 4-year survival interpretation

0–2 points:	80%
3–4 points:	67%
5–6 points:	57%
7–10 points:	18%

References

Association for Respiratory Technology & Physiology http://www.artp.org.uk/ (Accessed 7.12.2016).

British Thoracic Society (BTS) COPD consortium (2005). *Spirometry in practice.* https://www.brit-thoracic.org.uk/document-library/delivery-of-respiratory-care/spirometry/spirometry-in-practice/ (Accessed 28.11.2016).

Carter, R., Holiday, D.B., Nwasuruba, C., Stocks, J., Grothues, C. & Tiep, B. (2003). 6-minute walk work for assessment of functional capacity in patients with COPD. *CHEST Journal.* **123**(5), 1408–1415.

Celli, B.R., Cote, C.G. & Marin, J.M. *et al.* (2004). The body-mass index, airflow obstruction, dyspnea and exercise capacity index in chronic obstructive pulmonary disease. *New England Journal of Medicine.* **350**(10), 1005–1012.

Coakley, R. J., Taggart, C., O'Neill, S., & McElvaney, N. G. (2001). α1-Antitrypsin Deficiency: Biological answers to clinical questions. *The American Journal of the Medical Sciences.* **321**(1), 33–41.

Cooper, B. (2011). An update on contraindications for lung function testing. *Thorax.* http://thorax.bmj.com/content/early/2010/07/29/thx.2010.139881.full (Accessed 28.11.2016).

The European Lung Foundation http://www.europeanlung.org/en/ (Accessed 7.12.2016).

GOLD (2015). COPD diagnosis, management and prevention. https://www.guidelines.co.uk/gold/copd (Accessed 7.12.2016).

Kaufman, D. (2015). Interpretation of Arterial Blood Gases (ABGs). *Clinical education.* http://www.thoracic.org/professionals/clinical-resources/critical-care/clinical-education/abgs.php (Accessed 28.11.2016).

Kent, B. D., Mitchell, P. D., & McNicholas, W. T. (2011). Hypoxemia in patients with COPD: cause, effects, and disease progression. *International Journal of Chronic Obstructive Pulmonary Disease.* **6**(1), 199–208.

Leung, A.S., Chan, K.K., Sykes, K. & Chan, K.S. (2006). Reliability, validity, and responsiveness of a 2-min walk test to assess exercise capacity of COPD patients. *CHEST Journal.* **130**(1), 119–125.

Monso, E., Ruiz, J.,å Rosell, A. *et al.* (1995). Bacterial infection in chronic obstructive pulmonary disease. A study of stable and exacerbated outpatients using the protected specimen brush. *American Journal of Respiratory Critical Care Medicine.* **152**, 1316–1320.

Mims (2010). *Management of COPD (NICE Guideline).* http://www.mims.co.uk/management-copd-nice-guideline/respiratory-system/article/882159 (Accessed 28.11.2016).

NICE (2010). *Management of Chronic Obstructive Pulmonary Disease: Management of Adults in Primary and Secondary Care.* London: NICE. https://www.nice.org.uk/guidance/cg12 (Accessed 28.11.2016).

Pinto-Plata, V.M., Cote, C., Cabral, H., Taylor, J. & Celli, B.R. (2004). The 6-min walk distance: change over time and value as a predictor of survival in severe COPD. *European Respiratory Journal.* **23**(1), 28–33.

Polkey, M.I., Spruit, M.A., Edwards, L.D., Watkins, M.L., Pinto-Plata, V., Vestbo, J. & Coxson, H.O. (2013). Six-minute-walk test in chronic obstructive pulmonary disease: minimal clinically important difference for death or hospitalization. *American Journal of Respiratory and Critical Care Medicine.* **187**(4), 382–386.

Purves, W.K., Sadava, D., Orians, G.H., Heller, H.C. (2004). *Life: The Science of Biology.* 7th edn. Sunderland, Mass.: Sinauer Associates. p. 954.

Stockley, R.A., O'Brien, C., Pye, A., *et al.* (2000). Relationship of sputum color to nature and outpatient management of acute exacerbations of COPD. *Chest.* **117**, 1638–1645.

Turner, R., Angus, B., Handa, A. & Hatton, C. (2009). *Clinical Skills and Examination.* Oxford: Wiley-Blackwell Ltd.

Chapter 5

Acute conditions

This chapter will focus on acute presentations of respiratory disease. These are usually short-lived illnesses but can be life-threatening conditions. Patients may also go on to develop a chronic condition after an acute episode.

Some of the most common acute conditions affect the upper respiratory tract, including:

- Allergic rhinitis
- Congenital laryngeal stridor/laryngomalacia
- Croup – mainly a childhood illness
- Pharyngitis/Tonsillitis
- Epiglottitis
- Influenza
- Sinusitis
- Whooping cough (pertussis).

Lower respiratory tract diseases include:

- Acute bronchitis
- Bronchiolitis
- Pneumonia
- Respiratory syncytial virus
- Respiratory failure.

Acute bronchitis

Acute bronchitis is a self-limiting illness caused by a viral infection which leads to inflammation of the bronchial tubes. It is a commonly occurring illness, with approximately 5% of adults experiencing the condition each year (Macfarlane *et al.* 2001). It commonly lasts from a few days to 10 days but patients may continue coughing for several weeks post infection. It is commonly caused by influenza type A and B viruses, para-influenza virus, respiratory syncytial virus, coronavirus, adenovirus and rhinovirus and chlamydia pneumoniae (Hahn *et al.* 1991, Wenzel & Fowler 2006).

Influenza

The influenza season in the UK and the northern hemisphere is thought to be between December and March. Warmer weather has seen some earlier cases of influenza, although the predictive figures remain at the inter-seasonal state (Tappenden 2009, HPA 2013). Commonly known as flu, influenza is merely an inconvenience for a healthy individual, as it is a self-limiting disease from which people usually recover in 2–7 days. Influenza is classified as an RNA (ribonucleic) virus, from the *orthomyxoviridae* family, and is considered unstable, mainly due to the fact that the viral surface proteins haemagglutinin and neuraminidase keep evolving. New strains and variants are constantly emerging each year, particularly subtypes of influenza A and influenza B (PHE, 2013a). Pandemic influenza is thought to occur when a new type of influenza virus appears.

Transmission

The influenza virus is mainly transmitted from human to human by droplet spread, although there have been cases of animal to human transmission (WHO 2016). The incubation period is approximately three days, although nasal shedding can peak about 24–48 hours after onset of symptoms (Duncan 2013). Viral shedding starts within 24 hours before the onset of symptoms and continues for up to 5 days in healthy adults and 2 weeks in immunocompromised patients (Carral et al. 2008). It has also been shown that both influenza A and influenza B viruses can survive for 24–48 hours on hard, non-porous surfaces such as stainless steel and survive for less than 8–12 hours on products such as tissues (Bean et al. 1981).

Those at higher risk from flu include:

- The elderly, although the influenza vaccination may halve the incidence of serological and clinical influenza (Mangtani 2004)
- Children
- Pregnant women, who also have a depressed immunity and are therefore particularly vulnerable to severe complications of flu
- Those with chronic respiratory disease and particularly those who require continuous or repeated use of inhaled or systemic steroids or who have had a previous hospital admission because of an exacerbation (DH 2016)
- Patients with chronic cardiac, pulmonary, renal, hepatic or neurological disease or
- diabetes mellitus and a depressed immune system
- The morbidly obese (BMI > = 40).

Symptoms of uncomplicated influenza

Influenza is usually uncomplicated and these patients experience fever, coryza, malaise or myalgia, and sometimes have gastro-intestinal symptoms. Symptoms are:

- Fever or feeling feverish/chills

- A sudden temperature of 38°C (100.4°F) or above

- Cough

- Sore throat

- Runny or stuffy nose

- Muscle or body aches

- Headaches

- Fatigue (tiredness)

- Some people may also have vomiting and diarrhoea, though this is more common in children than adults (Dawood *et al.* 2009).

Treating uncomplicated influenza

Vaccination and prevention of spread is the key to eradicating this disease. Each autumn, however, there are more cases of influenza. The recommended treatment is as follows:

- Avoid dehydration by drinking plenty of fluids.

- Avoid visiting doctors' surgeries and hospitals where patients may infect other, more vulnerable people.

- Eat a healthy diet.

- Patients can self-administer the appropriate dose of paracetamol/ibuprofen-based painkillers or cold remedies to lower and regulate their temperature and relieve their symptoms. It is also advisable not to use aspirin to reduce the chances of developing **Reye's syndrome** (McGovern *et al.* 2001).

- Rest

- Stay at home to minimise spread

- Those in the 'at risk' categories should be treated with antiviral medication.

Influenza complications

- Patients with pre-existing respiratory conditions may experience exacerbations.

- Patients with chronic congestive heart failure may also experience a worsening of this condition, triggered by flu.

- Other non-respiratory complications may include: febrile convulsions, toxic shock syndrome, Reye's syndrome, **encephalopathy**, **transverse myelitis**, **pericarditis** and **myocarditis**.

- There is a high mortality rate affecting immunocompromised and healthy individuals (Rello & Pop-Vicas 2009, Rello *et al.* 2009).

Early warning signs are: decreased oxygen saturation, raised respiratory rate, diarrhoea, **hypotension**, elevated lactate dehydrogenase, creatine phosphokinase, and high creatinine levels.

Pneumonia

Every year, up to 480,000 adults develop pneumonia in the UK (NICE 2014b).

Pneumonia is the term we use when a patient has inflammatory consolidation of the lung tissue, and it can have viral, bacterial or fungal causes although it can also be due to chemical damage (Hull *et al.* 2009, pp. 152–153, Partridge 2006, p. 103). The lung tissue is damaged and loses its elasticity, as it is infiltrated by inflammatory **exudates**.

The most common causes of bacterial pneumonia are:

- Haemophilus influenza
- Mycoplasma pneumoniae
- Streptococcus pneumoniae
- Staphylococcus aureus.

The most common causes of viral pneumonia are:

- Adenovirus
- **Cytomegalovirus**
- Influenza types A and B.

Pneumonia is one of the most common infections in neonates and patients who are immunocompromised (Aly 2004). It is the term we use when a child has inflammation of the lungs and it can be due to viral or bacterial causes (Hull *et al.* 2009, pp. 152–153). It can be easily missed, as it presents with various signs and symptoms that make it difficult to diagnose at times. Signs can vary from lethargy and apnoea to poor appetite and jaundice. A raised temperature is another indicator that should be considered.

Adults may present with a variety of symptoms too. These are commonly breathlessness, cough, chest pain or discomfort, green **sputum** and fatigue. Signs can include **pyrexia**, **tachycardia** and **tachypnoea**. The signs of consolidation on chest examination are dull percussion notes, and additional signs (such as crackles, increased vocal **fremitus** and **whispering pectoriloquy**). The diagnosis can be confirmed on chest x-ray. Other possible tests may include a blood test for **C-reactive** protein (CRP) (NICE 2014b). Antibiotics are recommended if the CRP concentration is above 20mg/L (NICE 2014a). Microscopy is not routinely used to diagnose pneumonia unless there is a risk of moderate or severe community-acquired pneumonia (NICE 2014b). In these cases, you should consider using urine microscopy to identify Legionella pneumonia, and taking blood for further culture.

Treating pneumonia

The mainstay of treatment for bacterial pneumonia is the use of antibiotics. This is usually amoxicillin, macrolides or tetracyclines, depending on the type of bacteria involved. The recommended course is a single antibiotic for 5 days (NICE 2014a). Further supportive measures include medication for temperature control, rest and oxygen therapy for those with a low oxygen saturation level.

The community-acquired pneumonia (**CRB65**) score is a tool that can be used to assess the disease severity for community-acquired pneumonia (British Thoracic Society 2009). See Box 5.1 (below). Those with a score of 0 have a low risk of death. Those with a score of 2 or more should be admitted to hospital. The patient receives a point for each one of the following features:

- **C**onfusion
- **R**espiratory rate – 30 breaths per minute or greater
- **B**lood pressure – systolic of 90mmHg or less or a diastolic of 60mmHg or less
- **65** years of age or older.

Box 5.1: CURB65 score for mortality risk assessment

Give 1 point for each of the following:
- Confusion
- Raised respiratory rate
- Low blood pressure – a diastolic of 60mmHg or less.
- Age > = 65 years.

Score:

0 = low risk

1 or 2 = intermediate risk

3 or 4 = high risk.

Another tool is **CURB-65** or the CURB criteria. This is a clinical prediction rule that helps predict the mortality risk in community-acquired pneumonia. This tool has an additional assessment criterion (blood urea nitrogen level).

- **C**onfusion
- Blood **u**rea nitrogen greater than 7mmol/l (19mg/dL)
- **R**espiratory rate of 30 breaths per minute or greater
- **B**lood pressure less than 90mmHg systolic or diastolic blood pressure 60mmHg or less
- Age **65** or older.

Tuberculosis

Tuberculosis (TB) is caused by the bacteria mycobacterium tuberculosis and commonly occurs in the developing world (ERS 2016). The disease is transmitted from person to person, usually by droplet spread. Patients inhale droplets from those with active disease. Most people are carriers but only 10% of those who are infected go on to develop symptoms of the disease.

Diagnosing TB

The diagnosis of TB is based on personal history, clinical findings and the presence of tuberculi bacilli on hist8ology. Samples of sputum, urine, pleural fluid and cerebrospinal fluid can all be examined for the presence of acid or alcohol fast bacillus. Further tests may include chest x-rays and **bronchoscopy**.

Symptoms of TB

People can present with either pulmonary or extrapulmonary TB, and symptoms may appear several years after exposure to the bacteria. Common symptoms include: fever, haemoptysis, increased sputum production (with or without blood-stained sputum), night sweats, persistent cough and weight loss.

Preventing TB

The key to prevention is to vaccinate against the disease with the caccillus calmette-guerin vaccine (BCG). This is a live vaccine that is offered to children and those who are at high risk of catching the disease (PHE 2013). Until 2015 in the UK, the Heaf test was used prior to vaccination. This test requires patients to be injected with a purified protein derivative intradermally; and the response is then interpreted and graded. A response of grade 3–4 notifies the clinician that there is evidence of the disease, regardless of prior vaccination. For more information, please look at Chapter 32 of *Tuberculosis: the green book* (PHE 2013). However, the Mantoux test (or Mendel-Mantoux for purified protein derivative) is the most common worldwide TB screening tool.

Another important aspect of prevention is contact tracing. Anyone who has a confirmed case of TB will be asked to submit a list of people who may have been exposed to the disease through contact with them. The patient will need to be interviewed and a risk assessment carried out.

Treating TB

Treatment for tuberculosis is generally very effective and includes a multiple regime of four chemotherapic agents. It is important to note that there is an increase in multidrug-resistant TB which is resistant to isoniazid and rimfampicin, (ERS 2016). It is important to educate patients that their treatment therapy must be completed and often continues for six months. They may not begin to feel better for several weeks and even if they feel better they still need to complete the course of treatment.

Pleural effusion

This condition is defined as the presence of fluid between the visceral and parietal pleura. The patient may have an uncomplicated **pleural effusion**, where there is only fluid present, or a complicated pleural effusion. A complicated pleural effusion contains fluid that also has components relating to significant inflammation or infection. If left untreated, a complicated pleural effusion may become solid and create a constricting ring around the lung. This is a medical emergency. The effusion may contain serous fluid, pus, inflammatory cells or blood (in which case it is called a haemothorax).

Pleural effusions can develop when there is disruption of the formation and reabsorption of the pleural fluid. The main reasons for this are:

- An increase in the microvascular **hydrostatic pressure**
- A reduction in the pleural space pressure
- An ineffective **lymphatic system**
- A reduction in the vascular **oncotic pressure**.

Diagnosing pleural effusion

The presentation differs depending on the amount of accumulated fluid. When the fluid is more than 300mL, the patient can display clinical signs. Patients present with sharp acute pleuritic pain that gets worse during inspiration, a dry cough and increasing breathlessness.

Diagnosis is made on the basis of the clinical findings and secondary data. Percussion notes can be dull and tactile vocal fremitus may be absent. The top of the effusion may be auscultated, as breathe sounds can be diminished or absent. You may hear a **pleural rub** on auscultation.

A chest x-ray can indicate the size and position of the effusion. Further diagnostic tests include ultrasound and **computed tomography (CT) scanning**. These tests can give more accurate information about the size of the effusion and the underlying pathology.

Pleural aspiration can give the clinician an indication of the appearance of the pleural fluid and may also give the patient some relief. However, this procedure should not be performed if evidence points to a **transudate effusion** – unless patients demonstrate atypical features or they fail to respond to their treatment (British Thoracic Society 2010).

Pleural drainage is used to manage and treat an **empyema**, where there is a purulent pleural effusion. Drainage may result in:

- Straw-coloured fluid, which is normal pleural fluid
- Pink or red-stained effusion, which may indicate trauma or malignancy.

Pleural effusions can also be either transudate or exudate in nature, depending on the amount of protein present.

Transudate causes, in which the protein levels are < 30g per litre, may include:

- Cardiac failure
- Liver failure
- **Mitral stenosis**
- **Nephrotic syndrome**.

Exudate causes, in which the protein levels are > 30g per litre, include:

- Collagen disorders – **systemic lupus erythematosus (SLE)**
- Infective causes – TB

- Inflammation – secondary to **subphrenic abscess**
- Malignancy – commonly due to **mesothelioma** and breast cancer
- **Meig syndrome**
- Pulmonary infarct.

Secondary causes – secondary to infection.

Treating pleural effusion

The main aim of treatment is to identify the underlying cause of the pleural effusion. A small pleural effusion can be managed by observation and symptom relief. These patients can be discharged home with clear management instructions (British Thoracic Society 2010). However, patients with a large effusion and significant symptoms (such as breathlessness) will need hospitalisation and treatment.

Diagnostic aspiration is important if there is clinical uncertainty as to the type of effusion. The patient may need further chest drainage and antibiotic treatment, depending on the bacteria involved. Antibiotics are usually administered intravenously for speedy and effective treatment. Malignant effusions can also be diagnosed by pleural aspiration and cytology in about 60% of cases (British Thoracic Society 2010). Any question about the cause of the effusion should be thoroughly investigated by means of percutaneous pleural biopsy or bronchoscopy.

A **haemothorax** is commonly caused by trauma to the chest. It is diagnosed if the amount of **haematocrit** is 50% more than the amount in the bloodstream. Treatment includes the insertion of a large-lumen chest drain so that clots can be drained from the chest.

Pneumothorax

A **pneumothorax** can occur when air enters the pleural space either spontaneously or due to trauma. Spontaneous pneumothorax commonly occurs in thin young men in their early twenties (Partridge 2006). It is thought that the subpleural blebs and bullae, which are found at the lung apices, cause 90% of cases of spontaneous pneumothorax (MacDuff et al. 2010).

Presentation

The physical signs of a pneumothorax can be subtle and patients can complain of worsening symptoms over a few days (MacDuff et al. 2010). However, some patients may present with sudden acute breathlessness and pleuritic pain on the side of the pneumothorax. The symptoms directly correlate to the size of the pneumothorax. Patients commonly experience tachypnoea, tachycardia and **hypoxia**, and they can quickly deteriorate into a collapsed state and experience a cardiac arrest.

On examination, there may be a mediastinal shift with distended neck veins. Percussion will be resonant or hyper-resonant over the area of the pneumothorax, and a chest x-ray can help confirm this.

Treating a pneumothorax

Immediate emergency treatment includes inserting a chest drain to aspirate the air that is present in the pleural space. Patients may also need high-flow oxygen therapy to treat the hypoxia, although this needs to be carefully monitored. Most importantly, the clinician needs to determine the cause of the pneumothorax. Was it formed spontaneously? Or was it a secondary problem caused by an underlying lung disorder?

See the following link for an algorithm of care for spontaneous pneumothorax:
https://www.brit-thoracic.org.uk/document-library/clinical-information/pleural-disease/pleural-disease-guidelines-2010/appendix-3-spontaneous-pneumothorax-poster-pleural-disease-guideline/

Respiratory failure

Respiratory failure is a condition in which the arterial oxygen tension is less than 8kPa in air. The normal levels are 10–13kPa. There are two types of respiratory failure. Type I is when there is a PaO_2 less than 8kPa without hypercapnia. $PaCO_2$ can be normal or just below normal.

There is a reduction in the **alveoli** and capillary interface, which results in:

- Impaired alveolar gas exchange, which can be seen in cases of **chronic obstructive pulmonary disorder** (**COPD**), where there is destruction of the alveolar sacs. There may also be air-trapping, due to incomplete gaseous exchange. Pus or **mucus** can also damage the air sacs. In lung cancer, there can be damage to the lung **parenchyma**, reducing the number of alveoli.
- Thickening of the membrane.
- There is reduced capillary perfusion, which means:
- The arteries are obstructed, as in pulmonary emboli
- There is destruction of the pulmonary capillaries, as in COPD.

In Type II respiratory failure, the PaO_2 is less than 8kPa and hypercapnia is present. This is caused by impaired ventilation, in which patients cannot exhale CO_2. This can occur in any lung disease that is so severe that there is impaired gas exchange across the membrane (i.e. status asthmaticus).

Diagnosing respiratory failure

Patients can have a range of presentations, depending on the underlying cause of the respiratory failure. They generally have cyanosis, tachypnoea and signs of hypercapnia (see Box 5.2).

Box 5.2: Signs and symptoms of hypercapnia

- Bounding pulse
- Tachypnoea
- Dyspnoea
- Muscle twitching
- Warm extremities or flushed skin

- Tremor or flap
- Raised blood pressure
- Confusion
- Lethargy
- Headache.

Further diagnostic tests include:

- Arterial blood gases
- Pulse oximetry
- Imaging – chest x-ray or CT imaging
- Assessment of the diaphragm, such as phrenic nerve conduction tests.

Managing respiratory failure

The management of this condition includes assessing and determining the cause of the respiratory failure. Other aims include prevention of life-threatening hypoxia and hypercapnia. Patients may need oxygen therapy or invasive ventilation support (using an endotracheal tube), or non-invasive ventilation support (via a face mask).

Summary

This chapter has reviewed several acute conditions affecting the upper or lower respiratory systems. They all require immediate care and intervention by a healthcare professional. The acute conditions covered here include some of the conditions that are most commonly seen in an emergency department or at a doctor's practice.

References

Aly, H. (2004). Respiratory disorders in the newborn: identification and diagnosis. *Pediatrics in Review.* **25**(6), 201.

Bean, B., Moore, B. & Sterner, B. (1982). Survival of influenza viruses on environmental surfaces. *Journal of Infectious Diseases.* **146**(1), 47–51.

British Thoracic Society (BTS) (2009). Guidelines for the management of community acquired pneumonia in adults: update 2009. *Thorax.* **64**, 1–55s

British Thoracic Society (BTS) (2010). *BTS Pleural Disease Guideline 2010 – A Quick Reference Guide.* https://www.brit-thoracic.org.uk/document-library/clinical-information/pleural-disease/pleural-disease-guidelines-2010/pleural-disease-guideline-quick-reference-guide/ (Accessed 30.11.2016).

Carrat, F., Vergu, E. & Ferguson, N.M. (2008). Time lines of infection and disease in human influenza: a review of volunteer challenge studies. *American Journal of Epidemiology.* **167**(7), 775–785.

Dawood, F.S., Jain, S., Finelli, L. *et al.* (2009). Emergence of a novel swine-origin influenza A (H1N1) virus in humans. *New England Journal of Medicine.* **360**, 2605–2615.

Dirksen, A., Dijkman, J.H., Madsen, F., Stoel, B., Hutchison, D.C., Ulrik, C.S. & Vrooman, H.A. (1999). A randomized clinical trial of α1-antitrypsin augmentation therapy. *American Journal of Respiratory and Critical Care Medicine.* **160**(5), 1468–1472.

Department of Health (2016). *The national flu immunisation programme 2016–2017.* https://www.gov.uk/government/uploads/system/uploads/attachment_data/file/529954/Annual_flu_letter_2016_2017.pdf (Accessed 19.12.2016).

Duncan, D. (2013). Treatment and prevention of influenza. *Nurse Prescribing.* **11**(12).

European Respiratory Society (ERS) (2016). *Tuberculosis.* http://www.erswhitebook.org/chapters/tuberculosis/ (Accessed 30.11.2016).

Hahn, D.L., Dodge, R.W. & Golubjatnikov, R. (1991). Association of Chlamydia pneumoniae (strain TWAR) infection with wheezing, asthmatic bronchitis, and adult-onset asthma. *Journal of the American Medical Association.* **266**(2), 225–230.

Hull, J., Forton, J. & Thomson, A. (2009). *Paediatric Respiratory Medicine.* Oxford: Oxford University Press.

MacDuff, A., Arnold, A. & Harvey, J. (2010). Management of spontaneous pneumothorax: British Thoracic Society pleural disease guideline 2010. *Thorax.* **65**:ii18–ii31 http://thorax.bmj.com/content/65/Suppl_2/ii18.full.html (Accessed 30.11.2016).

Macfarlane, J., Holmes, W., Gard, P. *et al.* (2001). Prospective study of the incidence, aetiology and outcome of adult lower respiratory tract illness in the community. *Thorax.* **56**, 109–114.

Mangtani, P., Cumberland, P., Hodgson, C.R., Roberts, J.A., Cutts, F.T. & Hall, A.J. (2004). A cohort study of the effectiveness of influenza vaccine in older people, performed using the United Kingdom general practice research database. *Journal of Infectious Diseases.* **190**(1), 1–10.

McGovern, M.C., Glasgow, J.F.T. & Stewart, M.C. (2001). Reye's syndrome and aspirin: lest we forget. *British Medical Journal.* **322**(7302), 1591.

NICE (2014a). *More care should be taken when prescribing antibiotics for pneumonia.* Press release archive. https://www.nice.org.uk/news/press-and-media/more-care-should-be-taken-when-prescribing-antibiotics-for-pneumonia (Accessed 30.11.2016).

NICE (2014b). *Pneumonia in adults: diagnosis and management.* http://www.nice.org.uk/guidance/cg191/chapter/1-recommendations (Accessed 30.11.2016).

Partridge, M. (2006). *Understanding Respiratory Medicine.* London: CRC Press.

Public Health England. (2013a). *Surveillance of influenza and other respiratory viruses in the United Kingdom: Winter 2013/14* https://www.gov.uk/government/uploads/system/uploads/attachment_data/file/325203/Flu_annual_report_June_2014.pdf (Accessed 19.12.2016).

Public Health England (PHE) (2013b). *Tuberculosis: the green book.* Chapter 32. https://www.gov.uk/government/publications/tuberculosis-the-green-book-chapter-32 (Accessed 30.11.2016).

Rello, J. & Pop-Vicas, A. (2009). Clinical review: Primary Influenza viral pneumonia. *Critical Care.* **13**(6), 1.

Tappenden, P., Jackson, R. & Cooper, K. (2009). Amantadine, oseltamivir and zanamivir for the prophylaxis of influenza including a review of existing guidance no. 67): A systematic review and economic evaluation. *Health Technology Assessment.* **13**(11): iii, ix–xii, 1–246. doi:10.3310/hta13110

Wenzel, R.P. & Fowler III, A.A. (2006). Acute bronchitis. *New England Journal of Medicine.* **355**(20), 2125–2130.

World Health Organization (WHO) (2016). *Influenza.* http://www.who.int/topics/influenza/en/ (Accessed 19.12.2016).

Chapter 6

Chronic conditions

There are two main categories of chronic respiratory diseases: obstructive and restrictive disorders. Most of these diseases cause obstruction in the airways, due to narrowing of the smaller **bronchi** and larger **bronchioles**. This chapter will look at the two main obstructive diseases, **asthma** and **chronic obstructive pulmonary disorder** (**COPD**). Restrictive diseases are characterised by reduced lung volumes, due to an alteration in lung tissue or because of a disease of the **pleura** or chest wall, or neuromuscular processes. These conditions may have a significant impact on patients' morbidity and mortality.

Obstructive diseases

'Chronic respiratory diseases are a group of chronic diseases affecting the airways and the other structures of the lungs,' (WHO 2007, p. 12). These are asthma, COPD, **bronchiectasis**, hypersensitivity **pneumonia**, **lung fibrosis**, chronic pleural diseases, **pneumoconiosis**, **pulmonary eosinophilia**, **sarcoidosis** and sleep **apnoea** syndrome and cancer of the lung (WHO 2007, pp. 12–13). Two of these conditions, asthma and COPD, are very similar in presentation.

Asthma is a disease of the airways involving chronic inflammation, hypersensitivity of the airways and a variable airway flow (Fréour 1987, NICE 2012). It is similar to COPD because there is obstruction of air flow, often due to excessive secretion from the **mucus** glands and airway thickening due to scarring and inflammation. Unlike COPD, there is broncho-constriction, as the smooth muscle around the airways contracts. There is also bronchial inflammation that results in narrowing of the airways, due to **oedema** initiated by the immune response to **allergens**. Distinguishing between the two conditions can be difficult based on the clinical symptoms alone, especially in people over the age of 40 (Tinkleman et al. 2006). However, the clinician can distinguish between the two conditions, using a combination of history taking and spirometry testing (NICE 2011).

COPD

COPD is characterised as a chronic air flow limitation that is usually progressive and not fully reversible (GOLD 2016). It is also associated with an increased chronic inflammatory response in the airways to particularly harmful inhalants such as cigarette smoke (GOLD 2016). It is thought to be one of the major causes of worldwide mortality, sitting fourth in the league tables (GOLD 2016).

The World Health Organization (WHO) has predicted that COPD will become the fourth leading cause of death worldwide by 2030 (WHO 2007). In fact, it is expected to become the second leading cause of death within the next few years, as cases are increasing significantly. It is unclear whether this rise is due to more informed diagnosis or increased risks, such as an increase in cigarette smoking (Mannino et al. 2007).

A diagnosis of COPD should be considered in patients over the age of 35 who have a risk factor (usually smoking) and who present with one or more of the following symptoms: exertional breathlessness, chronic cough, regular **sputum** production and frequent winter 'bronchitis' wheeze (British Thoracic Society 2004). Although the main risk factor is smoking, this condition can also be due to passive smoking or pollution (British Thoracic Society 2004; Yin et al. 2007).

COPD is an overarching term that is used to describe a chronic disorder where there is air flow obstruction (NICE 2011). COPD has become a government priority since the Global Initiative of Obstructive Lung Disease (GOLD) was launched by the WHO, recognising COPD as a disease with a global impact (WHO 2010). However, COPD has been associated with poor morbidity since the 1950's, with the publication of Barach and Bickerman's book in 1956. Petty (2006) mentions that bronchitis has also been linked with COPD since at least 1944 by Ronald Christie in his book about it (Petty, 2006).

Fletcher et al. (1976) also identified the risk of smoking and COPD.

Box 6.1: Presentation of COPD

Patients with COPD usually present with:

- A persistent cough
- Progressive breathlessness
- Chronic productive cough
- Reduced exercise tolerance.

COPD is a major cause of morbidity and disability in the United Kingdom and it has been suggested that it will be the third-leading cause of death worldwide by 2020 (Murray & Lopez 1996). This is compounded by the fact that even when a patient presents to primary care with recognisable signs of the disease they are not diagnosed (Britton 2003). There are an estimated 2.7 million people who are undiagnosed (Idriss 2008). Under-diagnosis was also more pronounced in urban areas and is particularly severe in the Greater London area (Nacul et al. 2010). Ultimately, we can predict it will be in the top causes of morbidity and disease.

COPD is very similar to asthma in its presentation and physiology but management of the condition can differ (WHO 2007, p. 12). Asthma is a disease of the airways involving chronic inflammation, hypersensitivity of the airways and a variable airway flow, although the disease process is perhaps more complex than originally thought (Fervour 1987, Higashioto *el al.* 2015, NICE 2011). In the asthmatic airways, there is an increase in CD4+ **lymphocyte-, eosinophil-,** and **macrophages** during the inflammatory response (Kim & Rhee 2010, Woodruff *et al.* 2009). In COPD, inflammation is mainly due to the T-cell co-receptor CD8 glycoprotein and macrophages in the bronchioles and **alveoli** (Jeffery 1998, Kim & Rhee 2010, O'Shaughnessy *et al.* 1997.).

Asthma resembles COPD in that there is obstruction to air flow, and this is often due to over-secretion by the mucus glands and airway thickening caused by persistent inflammation. However, in asthma there is also broncho-constriction as the smooth muscle around the airways contracts. This bronchial narrowing can occur because there is an increase in **oedema**, initiated by the immune response to allergens. The inflammatory process affects the whole respiratory tract, from the larger to the small airways, in both COPD and asthma (van den Berge, 2011). The smaller airways are <2 mm in internal diameter. The thickness of the small airways can be assessed by measuring the forced expiratory flow rates at 50% of vital capacity (FEF 50%) and at 25% to 75% of vital capacity (FEF 25%–75%), and is a predictor of the severity of COPD (Bar-Yishay *et al.* 2003; GOLD, 2016; Hogg & Timens 2009).

Chronic obstructive pulmonary disease (COPD) is therefore characterised as a chronic air flow limitation that is usually progressive and differs from asthma in that it is not fully reversible (GOLD 2015). However, there has been increased discussion about how these separate diseases converge and this is known as Asthma–Chronic Obstructive Pulmonary Disease Overlap Syndrome (ACOS). ACOS occurs in 15–25% of obstructive airway diseases (Papaiwannou *et al.* 2014, Postma 2015). Some would define ACOS as a special phenotype of a spectrum of chronic obstructive airway diseases, in which asthma and COPD are polar opposites (Tho *et al.* 2015). Others would suggest that the inflammation associated with structural alterations of the large and small airways creates a transient phenotypic overlap (Kim & Rhee 2010). At present, there is no definitive description of ACOS (GOLD 2016).

The damage within the airways is thought to affect the small airways and lung **parenchyma**, (GOLD 2016). There is tissue fibrosis and smooth muscle hypertrophy (airway remodelling) in the small airways which results in **emphysema** (GOLD 2016). Clearly, COPD is not only a disease of air flow limitation but a complex heterogeneous disease (Agusti 2014).

Diagnosing COPD

Patients with COPD may present with bronchitic changes, emphysema or both. The three pathological changes that can occur in COPD are as follows:

- Loss of elasticity of the airways with destruction of the alveoli within the lung, resulting in loss of support and closure of small airways during expiration, as in emphysema (Postma & Rabe 2015).
- Narrowing of the small airways as a result of inflammation, tissue damage and loss of elastic fibres (Black *et al.* 2008).

- Obstruction of the lumen of small airways with mucous secretions. There are various inflammatory infiltrates in the mucous secretary apparatus, as in bronchitis (Posta & Rabe 2015). There is also hypersecretion of mucus, as there are goblet cells and enlarged submucosal glands due to chronic airway irritation (GOLD 2016). Pooling of the mucus can lead to increasing bouts of infection.

A diagnosis of COPD should be considered in any patient with a history of **dyspnoea**, chronic cough or sputum production but bear in mind that the diagnostic boundaries of respiratory disease often overlap. Other clinical features that are seen in severe disease are fatigue, weight loss and a low **body mass index** (**BMI**) (Celli et al. 2004). A low BMI should be considered as part of a scoring system such as BODE to predict prognosis, rather than as a stand-alone sign (Lainscak et al. 2011).

Spirometry is an important diagnostic test, as it can identify the presence of an obstructive pattern and the patient's post-bronchodilator FEV1. A FVC < 0.70 confirms the presence of persistent air flow limitation, which is a feature of COPD (GOLD 2016). Subjective data can be obtained using a simple measure of breathlessness, such as the Modified British Medical Research Council (mMRC) Questionnaire, to measure breathlessness although this only helps us measure one symptom of the disease (Bestall et al. 1999). There are also comprehensive disease-specific health-related quality of life or health status questionnaires such as the CRQ236 and SGRQ347. However, these are too long to use in practice.

Managing COPD

Every individual experiences a different pattern of disease and its debilitating symptoms. The management of a patient with COPD should therefore start with an individualised assessment of their current symptoms and future risks (GOLD 2016).

The aims of their care should be to:

- Improve their health status
- Empower the patient to self-manage their condition
- Prevent disease progression
- Prevent further exacerbation
- Reduce their symptoms
- Relieve their symptoms.

Smoking cessation

We know that smoking cessation is the major intervention that can improve the natural history of COPD (GOLD 2016). However, this is also the area of nursing and medical care that needs the most improvement (Stone et al. 2014, Tønnesen 2013). This is something that healthcare professionals need to focus on, as smoking cessation is the most effective intervention in stopping the progression of the disease, and can result in increased survival rates.

Perhaps, as nurses, we do not promote smoking cessation as much as we should in those patients with moderate or severe COPD, as we do not realise that it can make a significant difference. The rate of change in FEV1 is variable, with increased rates of decline among current smokers so smoking cessation therapies are helpful even in later disease (Vestbo et al. 2011). The risk of developing lung cancer and COPD increases if a patient continues smoking, and the risk also rises in relation to the number of cigarettes they smoke each day (Doll et al. 2004).

The most effective smoking cessation treatment for patients with COPD has been found to be counselling along with varenicline and nicotine replacement therapy (NRT) or bupropion SR (GOLD 2016). Patients with COPD found that this combination of intensive counselling and pharmacology was the most effective way of stopping smoking (Hoogendoorn et al. 2010).

Pharmacological options

There are a variety of pharmacological therapies for COPD but none has been shown to modify the long-term decline in lung function (GOLD 2016). Treatment should therefore focus on symptom relief for our patients. This includes the use of bronchodilators to offer symptomatic relief of breathlessness, whether they are **long-acting muscarinic agonists** (**LAMAs**), **long-acting beta2-agonists** (**LABAs**) or a combination of the two (GOLD 2016). First-line treatment should therefore be the combined use of short- or long-acting beta2-agonists (LABAs) with anticholinergics if symptoms do not improve with single agents (GOLD 2016, NICE 2015).

Inhaled corticosteroids (IHCs) have also been shown to reduce the number of COPD exacerbations and therefore improve the quality of life for patients but they cannot reduce the loss of lung function (Burge et al. 2000, GOLD 2016). There may also be an increase in the incidence of pneumonia for patients using IHCs.

Pulmonary rehabilitation

Pulmonary rehabilitation programmes usually include an educational component, which is beneficial for clients with COPD no matter how severe their condition. The educational component includes smoking cessation, an overview of COPD, self-management skills, management of exacerbations and discussion of end-of-life issues. Certainly, all patients who have persistent **shortness of breath** (**SOB**) on exercise should be offered pulmonary rehabilitation (Garrod et al. 2006). This type of rehabilitation has also been shown to improve anxiety and depression (Paz et al. 2007).

However, even though pulmonary rehabilitation has been shown to improve patients' exercise tolerance and dyspnoea, referral to this service appears to be sporadic – probably because it is offered to patients with moderate to severe COPD, as there is not enough funding available for a broad reaching service (Berry et al. 1999, Garrod et al. 2006, GOLD 2016).

There are also a range of mucus clearing respiratory devices such as an Acapella® or Flutter which use oscillating positive expiratory pressure to help your patient facilitate mucus clearance. A physiotherapist can instruct your patient how to use it as part of a breathing exercise regime.

Box 6.2: Reader activity

Find out what pulmonary rehabilitation services are available in your area. Ask if you can attend at least one session to find out more about what is involved.

Oxygen therapy

Oxygen therapy is delivered for patients who need emergency support, or short-burst or long-term oxygen therapy. Patients need to have a careful assessment, as inappropriate oxygen therapy may lead to respiratory depression (GOLD 2016, NICE 2010). This includes **full blood count** (**FBC**) test, **pulse oximetry** and **arterial blood gases** (**ABGs**).

Long-term oxygen therapy (LTOT), with continuous use of oxygen for 15 or more hours in a 24-hour period for patients with PaO_2 less than 7.3kPa, improves survival rates (Nott Group 1980, GOLD 2016). It also helps patients by alleviating symptoms and improves their health-related quality of life. Certainly, LTOT should be considered in patients with severe air flow obstruction (FEV1 30–49% predicted) (GOLD 2016).

Patients who have COPD and a PaO_2 less than 7.3kPa when stable, or a PaO_2 greater than 7.3 and less than 8kPa when stable, with one of the following – secondary polycythaemia, nocturnal hypoxaemia, peripheral oedema or pulmonary hypertension – should be on oxygen therapy (NICE 2010).

Short-burst oxygen therapy can be prescribed for the breathless patient, particularly during periods of exercise.

A holistic assessment of patients with COPD will identify areas in which they need nursing care and support. The main treatment options have been covered above, and any treatment should be tailored to meet the aims and objectives of good-quality care mentioned at the start of this section.

Alpha-1 antitrypsin (A1AT) deficiency

This is an inherited condition in which people lack the **alpha-1 antitrypsin** (**A1AT**) glycoprotein. There are several variants of the AAT gene. In A1AT the most important variants are S and Z, which are produced in the liver. There may be low levels of the protein (as it is still produced) but the A1AT molecule configuration is changed. It cannot be transported out of the liver into the bloodstream or passed onto the lungs. In severe cases, the accumulation of excess alpha-1 antitrypsin in the **hepatocytes** leads to destruction of these cells and therefore causes liver failure (Banauch et al. 2010). Other variants of the gene are: M, which is normal; S, in which low levels of AAT are produced; or Z, where very little ATT is produced. Patients can also have a combination of these variants.

The intrapulmonary Z alpha-1 antitrypsin also forms polymers, as in the liver but within the alveolar spaces. These act as a chemo-attractant for **neutrophils**. A1AT is particularly important in the lungs, where it mops up neutrophil **elastase**, thus preventing damage (Hill 2000, Lomas 2006).

This **enzyme** normally digests damaged or aging lung cells, foreign particles (including debris from smoking) and bacteria. Where there is a deficiency of AIAT, excessive inflammation occurs and progressive emphysema.

Patients with AIAT deficiency produce neutrophil elastase, which cannot be neutralised efficiently (Lomas 2006) and ends up destroying the alveoli in the lungs. As a result, the alveoli lose their elasticity, leaving them over-inflated and unable to expand and contract as normal. Holes also develop in their stretched walls, making them less able to fill with enough air and consequently even less effective. They may also develop air trapping.

This genetic disorder can be seen in neonates (causing neonatal **jaundice** and **hepatitis**) or in infants (as cholestatic jaundice). It can ultimately lead to hepatic cirrhosis or liver failure and is therefore the leading cause of liver transplantation in children.

If the disease mainly affects the lungs, non-smokers will usually present with the symptoms of emphysema in their fifties. Smokers may present up to ten years earlier, or may develop symptoms of dyspnoea in their thirties (Campos et al. 2005). Exposure to other environmental triggers may also speed up lung damage in patients with this disorder, as seen in members of the fire crews who attended the World Trade Center on 9.11.2001 (Banauch et al. 2010).

Management of AIAT deficiency is the same as that for a patient with COPD. Pharmacological management should include a step approach, starting with bronchodilator therapy (SIGN and British Thoracic Society 2011). Other forms of management are referral for pulmonary rehabilitation, education on diet and exercise and a yearly assessment of the patient and their ability to carry out self-management.

Genetic screening should also be considered for family members, as this is an inherited condition caused by a defective gene on chromosome 14 (also called the Serpina 1 gene). Everyone inherits two copies of chromosome 14. A normal person will be classified as PiMM, where Pi stands for protease inhibitor and M is the normal gene. There are over 70 variants where S and Z are the most common mutations of the alpha-1 antitrypsin gene. Patients can be affected by these genetic mutations or be carriers of them. Knowing whether they fall into either of these categories determines what treatment they should receive, and helps in disease prevention.

One controversial form of treatment is the use of intravenous (IV) augmentation therapy with alpha-1 antitrypsin, which is thought to benefit those patients with moderate obstruction (Chapman et al. 2009). However, a Cochrane review found that the evidence of efficacy was still not robust. The review relied heavily upon non-randomised studies of unknown quality, which made it difficult to confirm the reliability of the conclusions, even though a variety of studies were reviewed (Cochrane Library 2012). One organisation that is researching this therapy is the Antitrypsin Deficiency Assessment and Programme for Treatment (ADAPT) Group. This is based at the Bayer Lung Resource Centre in London.

Asthma

There are currently 5.4 million people with asthma in the UK – that is, 8% of adults and 20% of children (Asthma UK 2015). As mentioned previously, asthma is a chronic obstructive lung condition, which is often considered as a syndrome rather than a disease. It is a difficult syndrome to diagnose and is characterised by:

- Hyper-responsiveness of the airways
- Inflammation of the airways
- Reversible airway obstruction
- Typical symptoms of asthma, such as wheezing and coughing.

The diagnosis of asthma is based on clinical findings, as there are no succinct definitions of asthma and its types (British Thoracic Society 2014). Asthma is diagnosed based on symptoms, response to treatment and reversibility and spirometry. History taking also plays a vital part in the pre-diagnosis process of assessment. For instance, a patient may mention that their symptoms get worse when they enter a pet shop or during exercise; and history taking is particularly important if the client has occupational asthma.

Asthma is considered a disease of triggers, as exposure to these triggers precipitates the symptoms. An individual can inhale a number of different particles, and each one may trigger a reaction in which the muscle layer around the airway contracts, causing **bronchospasm** and production of mucus. The lumen of the airways also narrows and there is airway inflammation and hyper-responsiveness. This can cause narrowing in the airways, worsening symptoms and even lead to death. In 2014, 2016 people died from asthma attacks in the UK (Asthma UK 2015).

Aetiology of asthma

Asthma can be classified into two types. The first is atopic or extrinsic asthma, which is due to an allergy to particles that the airway is exposed to, such as house dust or pollen. The second type is called intrinsic or non-atopic asthma and this is due to secondary or recurrent infections of the bronchi and sinuses.

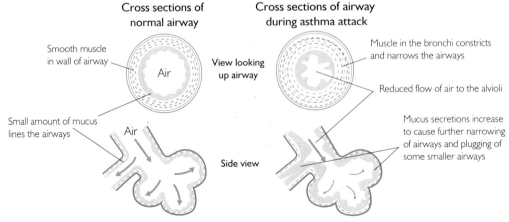

Figure 6.1: Asthma and the airways

The airways inflammation in asthma is caused by the **T-lymphocytes** and the action of the **interleukins**. In atopic asthma, mast cells link to IgE immunoglobulins, with the resulting release of mediators such as **histamine**.

In non-atopic asthma, local IgE immunoglobulins are released by the bronchial mucosa, and higher levels of **eosinophils** lead to the release of tissue-damaging proteins (see Chapter 1). The result is that structural changes occur in the airways from an early age. The basement membrane thickens and there are increased goblet cells producing an excess of mucus.

Diagnosing asthma

Once the differential diagnosis has been established, it can be confirmed using lung function tests. The gold standard test is spirometry with reversibility.

The normal symptoms of asthma are:

- Breathlessness
- Chest tightness
- Cough
- Sputum production
- Wheeze.

On examination, you may find evidence of atopic disease such as **eczema**. When examining the patient's chest, you may hear widespread wheeze on auscultation.

Reversibility testing

Reversibility testing involves assessing the FEV1 (or PEF) and/or symptoms before and after inhalation of 400 micrograms of salbutamol (British Thoracic Society 2014).

Treatment trials

If there is still diagnostic uncertainty and evidence of air flow obstruction or an incomplete response to inhaled salbutamol, then one can assess serial PEF recordings after a course of beclomethasone (200 micrograms twice daily equivalent for 6–8 weeks) or oral prednisolone (30mg once daily for 14 days).

For both these tests, a 400ml improvement response in FEV1 to either beta2-agonists or corticosteroid treatment trials will strongly suggest underlying asthma (British Thoracic Society 2014). However, there will be less of a response if patients have small airways disease or asthma/COPD overlap (Schermer et al. 2007). In rare cases, variables such as age and smoking history can also affect the results (Lehmann et al. 2006) and this is a reminder that the patient should always be assessed in a holistic manner. A diagnosis cannot be made on the basis of a test result alone.

In children, a diagnosis of asthma is based on assessment of symptoms, combined with family history and response to treatment (see Box 6.3 below).

Box 6.3: Diagnosis and the probability of asthma in children

Patients should have one or more of the following symptoms:

- Chest tightness
- Cough
- Difficulty breathing,
- Personal history of atopic disease.
- Response to treatment.
- Symptoms are worse at night and in the early morning
- Symptoms develop in response to specific triggers such as cold, pet dander, viral infections, emotions etc.
- Widespread wheeze heard on auscultation

Further tests

There are a few further tests that can be done:

- Chest x-ray – to exclude any other pathology in a newly diagnosed patient
- Total IgE levels can be tested, as these are elevated in atopic asthma; this is done by carrying out **radioallergosorbent testing** (**RAST**)
- A full blood count to assess the eosinophil levels, as they can be higher than normal in patients with atopic asthma
- Skin testing to identify specific triggers.

Occupational asthma

Occupational asthma is thought to be caused by the complex interactions of multiple genetic, environmental and behavioural influences, although a lot of these agents have been identified and the disease is categorised by the causative agent (Maestrelli et al. 2009). The specific workplace agents that cause allergic occupational asthma are recognised by the IgE-mediated mechanisms. These are generally high molecular weight compounds such as acid anhydrites, platinum salts, reactive dyes and sulfonechloramide. Other agents are isocyanates, persulphate salts, aldehydes and wood dust. Organic dusts (such as cotton or flax) can also cause asthma-like symptoms, though the aetiology of the disease is not yet fully understood (Dykewicz 2009, Maestrelli et al. 2009).

Aspirin sensitivity and asthma

The true prevalence of asthma related to sensitivity to aspirin or non-steroidal anti-inflammatory drugs (NSAIDs) is unknown, but this condition affects between 5% and 30% of asthmatics. Many do not develop the sensitivity until they are 30–50 years old, when symptoms of asthma and

sinusitis increase. People with these symptoms have also been found to have nasal **polyps** and chronic hyperplastic eosinophilic sinusitis (Stevenson 2009). Again, we are reminded of the importance of history taking.

Managing asthma

The aim of asthma management is to control the symptoms of asthma (British Thoracic Society 2014). With successful management, patients should have:

- No daytime symptoms
- No night-time awakening due to asthma
- No asthma attacks
- No exacerbations
- No limits to activity
- Minimal side effects from medication
- Normal lung function (FEV1 and/or PEF > 80% predicted or best).

To fulfil these aims, nurses should adopt a holistic approach to support their asthmatic patients. You may want to include complementary therapy, allergy avoidance, pharmacology and immunotherapy. Patients are also encouraged to self-manage their condition, with support from an asthma nurse, and make use of an action plan which outlines their management and what to do when. The next chapter will review these concepts in more detail.

Symptomatic asthma control is best assessed using the Royal College of Physicians (RCP) '3 questions' or the Asthma Control Questionnaire or Asthma Control Test (British Thoracic Society 2014, Thomas et al. 2009).

Table 6.1: The '3 questions' screening tool (adapted from the Royal College of Physicians)

In the last month:	Yes	No
Have you had difficulty sleeping because of your asthma symptoms (including cough)?		
Have you had your usual asthma symptoms during the day (e.g. cough, wheeze, chest tightness or breathlessness)?		
Has your asthma interfered with your usual activities (e.g. housework, work/school, etc.)?		

The interpretation of the above tool is:

- Answer no to all three questions = good control
- Yes to 2 or 3 questions = poor control
- Yes to 1 question indicates that there needs to be a more detailed questioning of the patient to assess their level of asthma control.

There are other tools you can use but this one seems to be particularly successful, especially in the community, and is the one recommended in the British Thoracic Society's guidelines (BTS 2014, Thomas *et al.* 2009).

Clearly, prevention of symptoms and early recognition of any deterioration are vital when managing asthma. Other key areas of asthma management are:

- Allergen avoidance
- Breastfeeding
- Pharmacological management.

Allergen avoidance

This process can start in early life to prevent sensitisation of the airways to specific allergens. The BTS (2014) guidelines do not recommend avoidance of potential allergens, such as house dust mites, in early life to prevent sensitisation of the airways to specific allergens, as the research in this area is not conclusive. They do, however, suggest avoidance of identified allergens. It is important to help patients identify their triggers, and support them to avoid these triggers or reduce their impact. An example would be to teach patients and their carers about damp dusting and regular hoovering of mattresses if they have an allergy to house dust mites. Specific guidance on this can be found on the _____ nces for further information).

_____ months has allergy-preventive effects for all infants, regardless of _____ ory of allergy (Sears *et al.* 2004).

Pharmacological management

A stepwise approach is used for the pharmacological management of asthma. This means that patients are started on the treatment level that is appropriate to the severity of their asthma. The aim is to control the symptoms as early as possible and step down medication whenever possible. The following adult summary is adapted from the BTS guidelines (2014). See also Figure 6.2.

- **Step 1 – mild or intermittent asthma:** Recommended treatment is the short-term use of short-acting beta agonists (bronchodilators) as required.

- **Step 2 – regular preventer therapy**: Start patients at a dose of inhaled corticosteroids appropriate to the severity of their disease. Titrate the dose to the lowest dose at which effective control is established. In adults, the starting dose of IHCs may be 400 micrograms of beclometasone dipropionate (BDP) equivalent per day. In children, the IHC dose may be 200mcg BDP per day.

- **Step 3 – add-on therapy**: Adults on IHCs at doses of 200–800mcg BDP/day, and children on IHCs at a dose of 400mcg/day, can be prescribed the following add-on therapies: 1. inhaled long-acting beta2-agonist (LABA); 2. a leukotriene receptor antagonist; 3. theophylline – the first choice as add-on therapy to inhaled corticosteroids in adults and children (5–12 years) is an inhaled long-acting beta2-agonist.

- **Step 4 – consider trial of IHCs 800mcg/day**. Increase to 2000mcg if that doesn't work. Add in inhaled long-acting beta agonist, theophylline or tablets slow release beta agonist. Refer to secondary care for advice and support.
- **Step 5 – high dose IHCs at 2000mcg/day**.

New treatments

There are always new developments in the treatment of these long-term conditions. One such medication, described as a 'game changer' for the treatment of persistent eosinophilic asthma', is Fevipiprant, a prostaglandin D2 receptor 2 antagonist (Worley 2016, Gonem *et al.* 2016). In Gonem *et al.*'s 2016 study, Fevipiprant caused a reduction in the mean sputum eosinophil percentage compared to the placebo group. It also had a good safety profile, with no serious adverse events reported during the study. The hope is that, after all the appropriate trials, it will be recognised by the UK Medicines and Healthcare Products Regulatory Agency and become part of our prescribing formulary.

Step 5: Continuous frequent use of steroids.
- Inhaled short-acting beta 2-agonist as required.
- High-dose IHCs (2000mcg/day)
- Use oral steroids at lowest amount for control.

Step 4: Persistent poor control.
- Consider trial of IHCs up to 2000mcg/day.
- Add in fourth medication such as a leukotriene receptor antagonist.

Step 3: Add-on therapy.
- Add on a long-acting beta agonist +/- and increase in inhaled corticosteroid.
- Trial of leukotriene receptor antagonist.
- Trial of slow-release theophylline.

Step 2: Regular prevention therapy.
- Inhaled corticosteroid.

Step 1: Mild/ intermittent asthma.
- Short-acting bronchodilators: inhaled short-acting beta2-agonists, as required.

Figure 6.2: Stepwise asthma management

Box 6.4 Asthma triggers

- Gender
- Emotions
- Laughter
- Crying
- Grass pollen
- Tree pollen
- Exercise
- Hormones
- Stress
- Viral infections
- Cold
- Heat
- Damp
- Pollution
- Mould and fungi
- Alcohol
- House dust mites
- Animals and pets
- Weather
- Smoking
- Change in season
- Non-steroidal anti-inflammatory drugs (NSAIDs)
- Beta receptor blockers
- Food preservatives and colourings such as monosodium glutamate

The following activity includes a case study. Please read the case study and consider what you think are the triggers for the patient. The answers to this activity are at the end of the chapter.

Box 6.4a: Reader activity – case study

Identify the asthma triggers in the following case study.

Janice is a 46-year-old woman who attends her local GP's surgery with a persistent night-time cough and fatigue. The practice nurse takes a full history from her and arranges for her to have spirometry with reversibility.

Family history: Sister has hay fever. Father died aged younger than 60 of cardiovascular disease.

Personal medical history: Asthma as a child. Recent hysterectomy for endometriosis. Anti-spasmodic for IBS. Hypertension.

Current medication: NSAID for pain relief. HRT. Beta blockers for hypertension.

Social: Lives in a detached house. Has recently moved to the countryside. Has two dogs and a cat. She has been stressed, as she is off work sick and her husband has recently been made redundant. They can just about afford the new house and, to make things worse, three weeks after moving in they discovered damp and mould in the upstairs bedrooms. She has tried to cope with the stress by increasing her exercise but that just makes the cough worse.

Restrictive lung disease

There are a range of diseases that have a restrictive pattern. The largest group are the interstitial lung diseases, also known as diffuse parenchymal lung disease. They can also be chronic or acute in nature. Diagnosis has become easier with more detailed **computed tomography (CT) scanning** and **bronchoscopy**.

Most of these diseases can cause a reduction or restriction in lung volume. They can be remembered by using the mnemonic PAINT: pleural, alveolar, interstitial, neuromuscular and thoracic cage abnormalities (Cariona & Brynd 2014). See Table 6.2. They may also be divided into two main groups based on the anatomical structures involved:

- Intrinsic lung diseases cause inflammation or scarring of the lung tissue or result in filling of the air spaces with exudate and debris. Examples of intrinsic lung disease include idiopathic fibrotic diseases, connective tissue diseases, drug-induced lung disease, and sarcoidosis.
- Extrinsic disorders involve the chest wall, pleura and respiratory muscles. Examples include non-muscular diseases of the chest wall and neuromuscular disorders.

Table 6.2: PAINT

Cause	Examples	Diagnosis
Pleural	Lung involvement, pleural scarring, large pleural effusions, chronic **empyema**, **asbestosis**	CT imaging, pleural biopsy, radiology
Alveolar	Oedema, haemorrhage	CT imaging, physical examination, radiology
Interstitial	Interstitial lung disease including idiopathic fibrotic diseases, connective tissue diseases, drug-induced lung disease, sarcoidosis	Echo, CT imaging, radiology
Neuromuscular	**Myasthenia gravis**, **amyotrophic lateral sclerosis (ALS)**, **myopathy**	Physical examination, blood tests
Thoracic/ extrathoracic	**Ascites**, **kyphoscoliosis**, pregnancy, obesity	Physical examination, secondary tests

Idiopathic pulmonary fibrosis

There are roughly 200 interstitial diseases, one of which is idiopathic pulmonary fibrosis. This is a debilitating lung disease that can occur in later life. There are few treatment options and mortality occurs within 3 years of onset (King *et al.* 2011, Raghu *et al.* 2011, Selman *et al.* 2004).

Aetiology of idiopathic pulmonary fibrosis

The condition is thought to be caused by abnormally activated alveolar **epithelial cells** which cause cell mediators to form fibroblast and myofibroblast foci through the mesenchymal cells. There is further attraction of circulating **fibrocytes** which also stimulated the epithelial to mesenchymal transition. The myofibroblasts produce large amounts of **collagen**, which destroy the lung architecture (King *et al.* 2011).

Signs and symptoms of idiopathic pulmonary fibrosis

- Patients present with cough, exertional dyspnoea, chest pain and a dry cough. They may also have finger clubbing and **cyanosis**.

- On chest examination, they may have basilar crackles.

- On spirometry, they have a restrictive pattern. Any patient with a restrictive pattern has to undergo further investigation. There is a honeycombing effect on CT scanning. Diagnosis is made based on CT scanning and histology (Selman *et al.* 2004).

Managing idiopathic pulmonary fibrosis

Immunosuppressant agent medication or tumour-blasting drugs such as interferon- 1b, pirfenidone, acetylcysteine, etanercept and bosentan have been trialled for this condition (Selman *et al.* 2004). The main aim of treatment is relief of symptoms and the final treatment option is a lung transplant (Lynch *et al.* 2007).

Sarcoidosis

This is the most common of the interstitial lung diseases and crosses all boundaries of race and gender, although it typically occurs in patients who are 20—40 years old.

Aetiology of sarcoidosis

This disease is characterised by non-caseating granulomas that grow in the affected organs. They are commonly found in the lungs or lymph nodes but can be found in a variety of places.

Signs and symptoms of sarcoidosis

There are a range of clinical signs and symptoms, partly depending on where the granulomas develop.

- In thoracic sarcoidosis, patients may initially present with no symptoms but can then go on to experience cough, dyspnoea, fever and malaise.
- On examination, they may have **erythema nodosum** and, in rarer cases, **finger clubbing**.
- On chest examination, the clinician may hear bilateral crackles on auscultation.
- On chest x-ray, there is bilateral hilar **lymphadenopathy**.

Managing sarcoidosis

Most patients only require symptomatic relief of their condition. It is only when there is organ involvement (such as the lungs) that treatment needs to be more aggressive. For more severe symptoms, steroid-sparing agents (such as azathioprine and methotrexate) can be used as alternatives. Immunosuppressant medications (such as cyclosporine or the anti-tumour necrosis factor treatment drug, infliximab) are also available. Studies with the selective phosphodiesterase 4 (PDE4) inhibitors, such as roflumilast, have been shown to have some success in treating sarcoidosis (Baughman *et al.* 2012).

Asbestosis

Asbestosis is a chronic lung disease caused by the inhalation of asbestos fibres. The main results of inhaling these fibres are pleural thickening and fibrosis as well as malignancy. Symptoms range from chronic severe shortness of breath to an increased risk of developing lung cancer.

Patients can initially present with a slow onset of shortness of breath, especially with physical activity (Sporn *et al.* 2004). On examination, the clinician may hear inspiratory crackles.

Diagnosing asbestosis

Diagnosis is made when there is:

- Visual imaging evidence of structural pathology consistent with asbestosis
- Evidence of causation by asbestos, as provided by the occupational and environmental history, and the presence of pleural plaques or asbestos bodies in the lungs
- The exclusion of other plausible causes for the findings.

An abnormal chest x-ray and/or CT scan remain the most important factors in establishing the presence of pulmonary fibrosis.

Pleural mesothelioma

Pleural mesothelioma is a type of cancer that is caused by inhaling asbestos fibres which affect the lining (or mesothelium) of the lungs. It can also cause pericardial or peritoneal mesothelioma.

The most common cause of mesothelioma is working with asbestos. Rare cases have been linked to talcum powder, irradiation of the chest and the simian virus 40 (SV 40). There is no conclusive evidence that these substances are the cause but they are thought to trigger the disease in clients who have also been exposed to asbestosis (Carbone *et al.* 1994, Broaddus & Robinson 2010).

The signs and symptoms include:

- Chest wall pain
- Pleural effusion, or fluid surrounding the lung
- Shortness of breath
- Fatigue or anaemia
- Wheezing, hoarseness or cough
- Blood in the sputum (**haemoptysis**)
- Presence of tumour on visual imaging.

Treating mesothelioma

Mesothelioma is a difficult disease to treat, with the mainstay of treatment being surgery, with or without radiation and symptom relief. Surgical resection of malignant pleural mesothelioma has been shown to have an 80% rate of local recurrence (Rusch *et al.* 2010). However, there have been some positive breakthroughs in this field, including the work of Dr Glen Reid, an associate professor at the University of Sydney Medical School, which uses a new drug delivery system that relies on nanotechnology and guiding antibodies (RT news 2015).

Bronchiectasis

Bronchiectasis is a chronic lung condition in which the walls of the bronchi are thickened, due to inflammation and infection. There is therefore abnormal airway dilation and poor mucous clearing of the airways. This causes pooling of the mucus and, as in COPD, patients can present with recurrent exacerbations or periods of infection. Both adults and children can have this condition. It may occur as a primary or a secondary condition, depending on the patient's past medical history.

A diagnosis should be considered when evaluating a child who presents with:

- A chronic moist/productive cough, especially between viral colds, or with positive bacterial cultures
- Asthma that does not respond to a variety of treatment options

- A single positive sputum culture for Staphylococcus aureus, Haemophilus influenza, Pseudomonas aeruginosa, non-tuberculous mycobacteria or Burkholderia cepacia complex
- An episode of severe pneumonia, particularly if there is incomplete resolution of symptoms, physical signs or radiological changes
- **Pertussis**-like illness, failing to resolve after 6 months
- Recurrent occurrences of pneumonia
- Persistent and unexplained physical signs or x-ray abnormalities
- Structural or functional disorders of the oesophagus and upper respiratory tract
- Unexplained haemoptysis
- Respiratory symptoms with any clinical features of **cystic fibrosis**, primary ciliary **dyskinesia** or immunodeficiency.

It should be considered in adults if they have:

- A persistent, productive cough
- Large volumes of very purulent sputum
- Pseudomonas aeruginosa
- Unexplained haemoptysis or non-productive cough.

Signs and symptoms of bronchiectasis

Symptoms tend to be the usual respiratory disease symptoms, such as dyspnoea, chronic cough, malaise and sputum production. The patient may have had a number of respiratory exacerbations in the last year. On general physical examination, you may find evidence of finger clubbing in 2–3% of patients, cyanosis and plethora with **polycythaemia**, reduced BMI, nasal polyps and signs of chronic sinusitis and even core pulmonale, in moderate to severe disease (Emmons 2015). On chest examination, there may be findings of persistent lung crackles, **rhonchi** and scattered wheezes on auscultation.

Secondary tests would include visual imaging such as chest x-ray and more detailed CT scanning, which should be standard imaging. Bronchoscopy and lavage would also be indicated to identify the cause of the infection (Emmons 2015, Tiddens 2006, Wilson et al. 1998). Other tests include serum alpha1-antitrypsin (AAT) levels to rule out AAT deficiency and COPD and Aspergillus levels. Vitamin D deficiency has been linked to bronchiectasis and Pseudomonas aeruginosa infections so these levels also need to be reviewed (Chalmers et al. 2013).

Treating bronchiectasis

The goals of therapy for bronchiectasis are to improve symptoms, to reduce complications, to prevent or manage exacerbations and to reduce morbidity and mortality. Antibiotic and airway clearance by chest physiotherapy are the main treatment options. First-line antibiotics for mild to moderately ill patients include a 7- to 10-day course of amoxicillin or a tetracycline. The newer macrolides, such as azithromycin or clarithromycin, have also been found to be effective in these patients (Davies & Wilson, 2004) and it is important to adhere to local prescribing guidelines.

Patients are taught to recognise the signs of a pending exacerbation or infection and treat it accordingly. It is recognised by WHO that self-management will ultimately lead to an improvement in this chronic condition (Epping-Jordan et al. 2004).

Lung cancer

This is the third most common cause of disease and the fastest-rising cause of cancer death this century. The main risk associated with lung cancer is smoking, which is thought to be the causative factor in 90% of cases. Smoking was identified as the foremost risk factor as early as the 1950s (Doll et al. 1950). Other risk factors include passive smoking, asbestosis and polycyclic hydrocarbons.

Prevention is therefore one of the main aims of management. The relative risk of lung cancer mortality also decreases following smoking cessation (compared with the risk associated with continuing to smoke). However, the lifelong increased risk in those who started smoking at a young age does not fall when smoking ceases, compared to the overall population (Cairns 2006). Certainly, the death rate falls in ex-smokers but that is mainly due to a reduction in cardiovascular and respiratory disease such as COPD.

Although there is no national screening programme, anyone who presents with a persistent cough for three weeks, breathlessness or blood streaks in their sputum should be assessed for lung cancer.

There are two main types of carcinoma of the lung: non-small cell carcinoma (NSCLC) and small cell carcinoma. This categorisation is based on the characteristics of the tumour cells at histology. This can also be used as a predictor of prognosis alongside gene expression profiles (Beer et al. 2002).

Small cell lung cancer

Small cell lung cancer (or oat cell cancer) accounts for 12% of all lung cancers. Commonly caused by smoking, it is a rapidly growing disease that responds well to chemotherapy.

NSCLC

There are three main types of NSCLC:

- Adenocarcinoma, the most common type of lung cancer: It develops in the mucous cells of the small bronchi. Patients may present with what appears to be consolidation or pleural effusion. On diagnosis, it is important to determine whether this is a primary or secondary type of cancer.

- Squamous cell, which develops in the epithelium of the large bronchi: It is often confined to the primary location. Patients may present with obstruction or haemoptysis.

- Large cell carcinoma, which is named after the large rounded cells visualised under a microscope: This type of lung cancer tends to grow quite quickly and therefore has a poor prognosis.

Signs and symptoms often occur in later disease. It is therefore important to assess a patient with any of these symptoms and rule out lung cancer as a potential diagnosis early in the process. Common signs and symptoms are listed below, and the most common ones are in italics:

- Bone pain
- *Chest pain*
- Clubbing
- Cough
- Dysphagia
- Dyspnoea
- *Haemoptysis*
- Hoarseness
- Stridor
- Unexplained weight loss
- Wheeze.

NSCLC investigations

Investigations would include spirometry testing, sputum culture and microscopy, taking a full blood count (including bone and liver biochemistry), cancer markers and visual imaging. Most tumours can be visualised on a plain chest x-ray. They may be present as a hilar mass or a lobar collapse.

Further tests would include bronchoscopy, transthoracic needle aspiration and biopsy.

Managing lung cancer

Management obviously varies depending on the type of lung cancer and the stage of the disease. Surgical management is offered to those with NSCLC and often involves a lung resection. Although this is unlikely to be curative, it can offer an increased life expectancy of five years or more. Chemotherapy is the treatment offered for small cell lung cancer, as the DNA of the cells is susceptible to the chemotherapy agents. Around 70% of patients respond to this treatment and survival rates for this disease are increasing.

Regrettably, many patients seek help when their disease is difficult to treat and their prognosis is poor. Early diagnosis is therefore important to reduce morbidity and mortality for this patient group. Smoking cessation and prevention remain key in the prevention of this disease.

Hyperventilation syndrome

Hyperventilation syndrome (HVS) can be separated into acute and chronic presentations. Acute HVS accounts for 1% of cases, in which between 10% and 30% of otherwise healthy individuals can present with chronic HVS (Duncan 2013). HVS is a disorder of breathing patterns with an unclear aetiology (Shu *et al.* 2007). It is thought to develop in childhood and is usually triggered by a traumatic event (Duncan 2013). HVS usually occurs between the ages of 15 and 55 years.

The signs and symptoms include:

- Chest pain
- Deep sighing
- Paresthesia: tingling in the extremities and around the mouth
- Panic attacks
- The patient breathes faster than normal, at a rate of more than 15 breaths a minute
- Yawning frequently.

Diagnosing HVS

Diagnosis is not straightforward, as many patients with hyperventilation syndrome do not have a low $PaCO_2$ during attacks. The diagnostic Nijmegen Questionnaire helps to provide an accurate diagnosis of hyperventilation if patients do not have triggering symptoms (Doorn *et al.* 1982, van Dixhoorn & Folgering 2015). Chronic HVS is certainly difficult to diagnose, as patients do not appear to be over-breathing and can present with a myriad of respiratory, cardiac, neurological or gastrointestinal symptoms.

Treating HVS

Patients with HVS can be referred to mental health services for treatment by a psychiatrist, psychologist or family physician. They can also be seen by physiotherapists with experience in retraining patients using proper breathing techniques.

Summary

As we have seen, there are several chronic respiratory conditions which are classified as restrictive or obstructive diseases. They can be debilitating and frustrating for our patients and their families. However, if patients are informed about their condition and are aware of the treatment options, they can learn to self-manage their disease. The next chapter will look at self-management in more depth.

Box 6.5b: Answers to reader activity

The asthma triggers are as follows:

- Gender
- Hormonal

- NSAID
- Beta blocker
- Pets
- Pollens
- Stress
- Fungi/mould
- Exercise.

Resources

More information about asthma:
https://www.asthma.org.uk/about/media/facts-and-statistics/

More information about bronchiectasis and self-management:
http://www.bronchiectasishelp.org.uk/#features/3

More information about mesothelioma:
http://www.mesotheliomaguide.com/

References

Aly, H. (2004). Respiratory disorders in the newborn. *Paediatrics in Review.* **25**(6), 201.

Asthma UK (2015). *Facts and statistics.* https://www.asthma.org.uk/about/media/facts-and-statistics/ (Accessed 2.12.2016).

Barach, A.L. & Bickerman, H.A. (eds) (1956). *Pulmonary Emphysema.* Baltimore: Williams & Wilkins.

Bar-Yishay, E., Amirav, I. & Goldberg, S. (2003). Comparison of maximal midexpiratory flow rate and forced expiratory flow at 50% of vital capacity in children. *Chest.* **123**(3), 731–735.

Baughman, R.P., Judson, M.A., Ingledue, R. et al. (2012). Efficacy and safety of apremilast in chronic cutaneous sarcoidosis (PDF). *Archives of Dermatology.* **148** (2), 262–264.

Beer, D.G., Kardia, S.L., Huang, C.C., Giordano, T.J., Levin, A.M., Misek, D.E. & Lizyness, M.L. (2002). Gene-expression profiles predict survival of patients with lung adenocarcinoma. *Nature Medicine.* **8**(8), 816–824.

Britton, M. (2003). The burden of COPD in the UK: results from the Confronting COPD survey. *Respiratory Medicine.* **97**, S71–S79.

British Thoracic Society (BTS) (2014). SIGN 141. *British guidelines on the management of asthma.* https://www.brit-thoracic.org.uk/document-library/clinical-information/asthma/btssign-asthma-guideline-2014/ (Accessed 2.12.2016).

Broaddus, V. C. & Robinson, B.W.S. (2010). Chapter 75. *Murray & Nadel's Textbook of Respiratory Medicine.* 5th edn. Philadelphia: Saunders Elsevier.

Cairns, J. (2006). Cancer and the immortal strand hypothesis. *Genetics.* **174**, 1069–1072.

Carbone, M., Pass, H. I., Rizzo, P., Marinetti, M., Di Muzio, M., Mew, D.J. & Procopio, A. (1994). Simian virus 40-like DNA sequences in human pleural mesothelioma. *Oncogene.* **9**(6), 1781–1790.

Caronia, J. & Byrd, R. (2014). Restrictive Lung Disease. *Medscape.* http://emedicine.medscape.com/article/301760-overview (Accessed 2.12.2016).

Chalmers, J.D., McHugh, B.J., Docherty, C., Govan, J.R. & Hill, A.T. (2013). Vitamin-D deficiency is associated with chronic bacterial colonisation and disease severity in bronchiectasis. *Thorax.* **68**(1), 39–47.

Davies, G. & Wilson, R. (2004). Prophylactic antibiotic treatment of bronchiectasis with azithromycin. *Thorax.* **59**(6), 540–541.

Doorn, P.V., Folgering, H.T.M. & Colla P. (1982). Control of the end-tidal PCO_2 in the hyperventilation syndrome: effects of biofeedback and breathing instructions compared. *Bulletin of European Physiopathology and Respiration.* **18**, 829–836.

Dykewicz, M.S. (2009). Occupational asthma: current concepts in pathogenesis, diagnosis, and management. *Journal of Allergy and Clinical Immunology.* **123**(3), 519–528.

Doll, R. & Hill, A.B. (1950). Smoking and carcinoma of the lung. *British Medical Journal.* **221**(ii), 739–48.

Emmons, E. (2015). Bronchiectasis. *Medscape.* http://emedicine.medscape.com/article/296961-overview (Accessed 2.12.2016).

Epping-Jordan, J.E., Pruitt, S.D., Bengoa, R. & Wagner, E.H. (2004). Improving the quality of health care for chronic conditions. *Quality and Safety in Health Care.* **13**, 299–305.

European Respiratory Society. *European Lung White Book.* http://www.erswhitebook.org/chapters/occupational-risk-factors/ (Accessed 2.12.2016).

Fletcher, C.M., Peto, R., Tinker, C.M. & Speizer, F.E. (1976). *The Natural History of Chronic Bronchitis and Emphysema.* Oxford: Oxford University Press.

Fréour, P. (1987). Definition of asthma. *CHEST Journal.* **91**(6_Supplement), 191S–192S.

Global Initiative for Chronic Obstructive Lung Disease (GOLD). (2016). *Global Strategy for Diagnosis, Management, and Prevention of COPD.* http://www.goldcopd.org/global-strategy-diagnosis-management-prevention-copd-2016/ (Accessed 3.12.2016).

Gonem, S., Berair, R., Singapuri, A., Hartley, R., Laurencin, M.F., Bacher, G. & Mansur, A.H. (2016). Fevipiprant, a prostaglandin D 2 receptor 2 antagonist, in patients with persistent eosinophilic asthma: a single-centre, randomised, double-blind, parallel-group, placebo-controlled trial. *The Lancet Respiratory Medicine.* **4**(9), 699–707.

Higashimoto, Y., Honda, N., Yamagata, T., Sano, A., Nishiyama, O., Sano, H. & Tohda, Y. (2015). Exertional dyspnoea and cortical oxygenation in patients with COPD. *European Respiratory Journal.* ERJ–00541.

Hogg, J.C. & Timens, W. (2009). The pathology of chronic obstructive pulmonary disease. *Annual Review of Pathological Mechanical Disease*. **4**, 435–459.

Hoogendoorn, M., Feenstra, T.L., Hoogenveen, R.T. & Rutten-van Mölken, M.P. (2010). Long-term effectiveness and cost-effectiveness of smoking cessation interventions in patients with COPD. *Thorax*. **65**(8), 711–718.

Kim, S.R. & Rhee, Y.K. (2010). Overlap between asthma and COPD: where the two diseases converge. *Allergy, Asthma and Immunology Research*. **2**(4), 209–214.

King, T.E., Pardo, A. & Selman, M. (2011). Idiopathic pulmonary fibrosis. *The Lancet*. **378**(9807), 1949–1961.

Lehmann, S., Bakke, P.S., Eide, G.E., Humerfelt, S. & Gulsvik, A. (2006). Bronchodilator reversibility testing in an adult general population; the importance of smoking and anthropometrical variables on the response to a β2-agonist. *Pulmonary Pharmacology and Therapeutics*. **19**(4), 272–280.

Lynch, J.P., Fishbein, M.C., Saggar, R., Zisman, D.A. & Belperio, J.A. (2007). Idiopathic pulmonary fibrosis. *Expert Review of Respiratory Medicine*. **1**(3), 377–389.

Maestrelli, P., Boschetto, P., Fabbri, L.M. & Mapp, C.E. (2009). Mechanisms of occupational asthma. *Journal of Allergy and Clinical Immunology*. **123**(3), 531–542.

Mannino, D.M. & Buist, A.S. (2007). Global burden of COPD: risk factors, prevalence, and future trends. *The Lancet*. **370**(9589), 765–773.

Murray, C.J., Lopez, A.D., Mathers, C.D. & Stein, C. (2001). *The Global Burden of Disease 2000 project: aims, methods and data sources*. http://www.who.int/healthinfo/paper36.pdf (Accessed 19/12/2016).

Nacul, L., Soljak, M., Samarasundera, E., Hopkinson, N.S., Lacerda, E., Indulkar, T. & Majeed, A. (2010). COPD in England: a comparison of expected, model-based prevalence and observed prevalence from general practice data. *Journal of Public Health*. fdq031.

NICE (2011). *Chronic obstructive pulmonary disease in adults*. http://www.nice.org.uk/guidance/qs10 (Accessed 14/12/2016).

NOTT group (1980). Continuous or nocturnal oxygen therapy in hypoxaemic chronic obstructive lung disease: a clinical trial. *Annals of Internal Medicine*. **93**, 391–398

O'Shaughnessy, T.C., Ansari, T.W., Barnes, N.C., & Jeffery, P. K. (1997). Inflammation in bronchial biopsies of subjects with chronic bronchitis: inverse relationship of CD8+ T lymphocytes with FEV1. *American Journal of Respiratory and Critical Care Medicine*. **155**(3), 852–857.

Paz, D., de Montes, O., López, J. et al. (2007). Pulmonary rehabilitation improves depression, anxiety, dyspnoea and health status in patients with COPD. *American Journal of Physical Medicine & Rehabilitation*. 86, 30–36.

Petty, T. (2006). The history of COPD. *International Journal of COPD*. **1**(1), 3–14.

Raghu, G., Collard, H.R., Egan, J.J. et al. (2011). An official ATS/ERS/JRS/ALAT statement: Idiopathic pulmonary fibrosis: Evidence-based guidelines for diagnosis and management. *American Journal of Respiratory and Critical Care Medicine*. 183(6), 788–824.

Rusch, V.W., Piantadosi, S. & Holmes, E.C. (1991). The role of extrapleural pneumonectomy in malignant pleural mesothelioma. A Lung Cancer Study Group trial. *The Journal of Thoracic and Cardiovascular Surgery*. **102**(1), 1–9.

RT news (2015). Groundbreaking cure for deadly asbestos-related cancer could be near. https://www.rt.com/news/267172-asbestos-mesothelioma-cancer-treatment/ (Accessed 2.12.2016).

Schermer, T., Heijdra, Y., Zadel, S., van den Bemt, L., Boonman-de Winter, L., Dekhuijzen, R. & Smeele, I. (2007). Flow and volume responses after routine salbutamol reversibility testing in mild to very severe COPD. *Respiratory Medicine*. **101**(6), 1355–1362.

Sears, M.R., Greene, J.M., Willan, A.R., Taylor, D.R., Flannery, E.M., Cowan, J.O. et al. (2002). Long-term relation between breastfeeding and development of atopy and asthma in children and young adults: a longitudinal study. *Lancet*. **360**(9337), 901–907.

Selman, M., Thannickal, V.J., Pardo, A., Zisman, D.A., Martinez, F.J. & Lynch, I.J.P. (2004). Idiopathic pulmonary fibrosis. *Drugs*. **64**(4), 405–430.

Shu, B.C., Chang, Y.Y., Lee, F.Y. et al. (2007). Parental attachment, premorbid personality, and mental health in young males with hyperventilation syndrome. *Psychiatry Research*. **153**(2), 163–170.

Sporn, T.A., Roggli, V.L. & Oury, T.D. (2004). *Pathology of asbestos-associated diseases*. Berlin: Springer.

Stevenson, D.D. (2009). Aspirin sensitivity and desensitization for asthma and sinusitis. *Current Allergy and Asthma Reports*. **9**(2), 155–163.

Thomas, M., Gruffydd-Jones, K., Stonham, C., Ward, S. & Macfarlane, T.V. (2009). Assessing asthma control in routine clinical practice: use of the Royal College of Physicians' '3 Questions'. *Primary Care Respiratory Journal*. **18**(2), 83–88.

Tiddens, H.A. (2006). Chest computed tomography scans should be considered as a routine investigation in cystic fibrosis. *Paediatric Respiratory Review*. **7**(3), 202–208.

Tinkelman, D. G., Price, D. B., Nordyke, R. J., & Halbert, R. J. (2006). Misdiagnosis of COPD and asthma in primary care patients 40 years of age and over. *Journal of Asthma*. **43**(1), 75–80.

Tønnesen, P. (2013). Smoking cessation and COPD. *European Respiratory Review*. **22**(127), 37–43.

Yin, P., Jiang, C.Q., Cheng, K.K., Lam, T.H., Lam, K.H., Miller, M.R. & Adab, P. (2007). Passive smoking exposure and risk of COPD among adults in China: the Guangzhou Biobank Cohort Study. *The Lancet*. **370**(9589), 751–757.

Van den Berge, M., ten Hacken, N.H., Cohen, J., Douma, W.R. & Postma, D.S. (2011). Small airway disease in asthma and COPD: clinical implications. *CHEST Journal*. **139**(2), 412–423.

van Dixhoorn, J. & Folgering, H. (2015). The Nijmegen Questionnaire and dysfunctional breathing. *ERJ Open Research*. **1**(1), 00001–2015.

Vestbo, J., Hurd, S.S., Agustí, A.G. et al. (2013). Global strategy for the diagnosis, management, and prevention of chronic obstructive pulmonary disease: GOLD executive summary. *American Journal of Respiratory Critical Care Medicine*. **187**(4), 347–365.

Wilson, C.B., Jones, P.W., O'Leary, C.J. et al. (1998). Systemic markers of inflammation in stable bronchiectasis. *European Respiratory Journal*. **12**, 820–824.

Woodruff, P.G., Modrek, B., Choy, D.F., Jia, G., Abbas, A.R., Ellwanger, A. & Fahy, J.V. (2009). T-helper type 2–driven inflammation defines major subphenotypes of asthma. *American Journal of Respiratory and Critical Care Medicine*. **180**(5), 388–395.

World Health Organization (WHO) (2007). *Living with chronic lung diseases*. http://tinyurl.com/z5csbul (Accessed 13/12/2016).

Worley, W. (2016). Asthma pill could prove "game changer" for people with severe symptoms. *Independent*. http://www.independent.co.uk/news/science/archaeology/news/asthma-pill-game-changer-fevipiprant-severe-forms-respiratory-condition-a7175981.html (Accessed 13/12/2016).

Chapter 7

Self-management

In this chapter, we will look at the importance of medical adherence. The aims of treatment for patients with respiratory disease are: reducing symptoms, preventing exacerbations and delaying the progression of the disease through the use of medication (GOLD 2016).

Medication can give immediate life-saving relief for some individuals with respiratory disease. However, in some cases, such as patients with chronic obstructive pulmonary disorder (COPD), medication has not been shown to modify the long-term decline of lung function. Nevertheless, there are various effective medications available to prevent and control symptoms, improving patients' health status, and reducing the occurrence of COPD exacerbations within the framework of self-management (GOLD 2008, GOLD 2016, Pauwels *et al.* 2001). Although some medications have been shown to be effective, it is not always possible to determine how effective they are, as about 50% of patients do not take their medications as prescribed (Brown & Bussell 2011).

Box 7.1a: Reader activity

List five reasons why you think people do not take their medication as prescribed.

Some suggested answers are at the end of the chapter.

Non-adherence has been shown to be a significant risk factor for mortality, morbidity, hospital admission and increased mortality (Rand 2005). Patient adherence to medication is known to be poor – and more so for COPD compared with other long-term conditions (DiMatteo *et al.* 2002, George *et al.* 2007).

Medication review

Embedded in the standard annual review for patients with long-term respiratory disease is the review of a patient's inhaler technique. Only around 1 out of 10 patients with a **metered dose inhaler**

(**MDI**) use the correct technique (Restrepo et al. 2008). Hesselink et al. (2001), suggest this can be as high as 100% for patients using inhaler devices. Educating patients about their inhaler device will therefore improve their technique. We have known for over a decade that understanding about inhaler devices and how they work improves adherence (Bourbeau & Bartlett 2008, Molimard 2005). This makes a difference to their medication control but there also needs to be a review of their medical adherence, which includes reviewing their daily dosing frequency (Toy et al. 2011).

Medication adherence

Non-adherence to medication has a significant effect on the patient's physical condition because they are not taking medication that may help reduce their symptoms. Non-adherence also has a significant impact on an already over-stretched NHS, as there are increased costs due to rising healthcare utilisation such as frequent attendance at A&E or referrals to secondary care (Golay 2011, Toy et al., van Boven et al. 2014). Costs can also be related to unused medication or its disposal, or to lost productivity due to sick days taken off work.

The other aspect to be considered is the cost to the patient. Many patients with long-term conditions will cut back on medication to save money if they are not eligible for free prescriptions or cannot afford a pre-paid prescription card (Egred et al. 2005, Piette et al. 2004). These patients may not take their medication simply because they cannot afford it.

Treatment adherence

Adherence to treatment is defined by the World Health Organization (2003) as 'the extent to which a person's behaviour corresponds with the agreed recommendations from a healthcare provider'. Meanwhile, Haynes et al. (1979) defined adherence in a more detailed way, as 'the extent to which a person's behaviour (in terms of taking medications, following diets, or executing lifestyle changes) coincides with medical or health advice'.

Non-adherence and adherence are difficult concepts to measure because we are asking whether or not the patient is utilising their prescribed medication. Generally, adherence is measured using subjective measures such as self-reporting and objective measures such as electronic prescription requests (Mäkelä et al. 2013). Patients who adhere to medical therapy generally tend to be older and from a high socio-economic group. They are usually better educated, have a stable lifestyle, and attend their outpatient appointments regularly (Lareau et al. 2010, Turner et al. 1995).

Medication adherence in respiratory disease

Under-use is one of the most common types of poor adherence to therapy (Dompeling et al. 1992, Hatton et al. 1996) and COPD patients have been shown to have a lower adherence to treatment than patients with **asthma** (Cochrane 1992). Over-use has also been shown to be an inappropriate use of medication (Dolce et al. 1991, Pepin et al. 1996) and this is the most common type of non-adherence in patients with COPD (George et al. 2005). In fact, Restrepo et al. (2008) suggest that only an average of 40%–60% of patients with COPD adhere to their prescribed regimen.

The reasons for non-adherence

The reasons for non-adherence seem to be very varied, ranging from lack of patient knowledge about their condition to anxieties about the medication's side effects. These reasons seem to be the same for asthma and COPD (Mäkelä et al. 2013).

The relationship between medication adherence and **health-related quality of life (HRQOL)** is well documented (Ágh et al. 2013, Ágh et al. 2014). If a patient is aware of the effectiveness of their medication, they will continue taking it. However, if there are side effects or social stigma that affect their HRQOL, they may not take their medication as prescribed. The side effects of the medication, and the social stigma caused by the treatment, may be more significant for the patient than the beneficial effects of taking the medication (Ágh et al. 2013).

Stigmatisation and lack of understanding about the disease appear to be particularly significant concerns for those with respiratory disease (Berger et al. 2010, Johnson et al. 2007). They may be afraid to take their medication because they are worried about what people may think of them while they are taking it. This fear may be partly linked to the fact that the main cause of COPD is smoking (Berger et al. 2010, Johnson et al. 2007).

There are certainly several factors that can affect a patient's medical adherence. These are listed in Table 7.1 (below).

Table 7.1: Factors affecting medical adherence
(adapted from The Global Initiative for Asthma (GINA) 2011, http://ginasthma.org)

Pharmacological factors	Non-pharmacological factors
Difficulties with inhaler devices	Lack of knowledge or instruction
Complex medication regimens	Lack of knowledge and/or understanding about the disease
Side effects	Inappropriate expectations
Anxiety related to side effects	Denial about the condition
Complacency	Lack of trust in healthcare professionals
Stigmatisation	Cultural/health beliefs

Strategies to reduce non-adherence

Various strategies can be used to increase patient adherence. These range from the use of self-management to simpler dosing regimens. Clinicians can play a critical role in helping patients with COPD understand their disease and the benefits of treatment, and in helping patients address their anxieties about potential side effects and supporting them to develop self-management skills (Bourbeau & Bartlett 2008). The barriers to medication adherence are complex and may differ from patient to patient. Solutions to improve medication adherence therefore need to be multifactorial (Brown & Bussell 2011).

Self-management and adherence

Self-management has been shown to improve health outcomes, leading to fewer hospital admissions. Patients report they have greater confidence and reduced anxiety about managing their condition (Challis et al. 2010, Purdy 2012). It has also been shown to improve adherence to treatment and medication (Challis et al. 2010). The educational programme offered should be tailored to the condition, with an action plan for the patient to use if they have an event such as a period of exacerbation (Da Silva 2011).

Self-management with adherence to an action plan is associated with a reduction in exacerbation recovery time (Bischoff et al. 2011, Lareau & Yawn 2010). Tailoring the self-management and action plan to fit the individual's needs, educational ability and capabilities seems to be a key component in effective self-management (Dowson et al. 2004). This can best be accomplished by enabling patients to be active participants in treatment decisions (Lareau & Yawn 2010). Certainly, the educational and self-management principles discussed in pulmonary rehabilitation mitigate the patient's experience of stigma and empower them to control their condition effectively (Partridge 2004).

However, Rice et al. (2010) suggest that effective pulmonary rehabilitation requires a more complex programme than that outlined by Walters et al. (2010). They suggest that patients should have education sessions, a personalised action plan (particularly for self-treatment of exacerbation), and monthly follow-up calls from a case manager, rather than one session of education and an action plan. The latter often occurs in general practice, as practice nurses frequently instigate the patient's action plan with a single education session. I am not suggesting that we should not give action plans to our patients, as we know that adherence to an action plan is associated with a reduction in exacerbation recovery time (Bischoff et al. 2011). There is also an increase in adherence to any medication intervention if it is part of a fuller educational programme.

Furthermore, there needs to be effective communication between the patient and their care provider about how the patient can implement these principles (Lareau & Yawn 2010). For instance, patients may have concerns about when to take their medication or its side effects. If there is open and effective communication, they can express these concerns and together the clinician and patient can determine a plan best suited to the patient. Patients also appear to be more concordant and adherent to their medication if they are actively involved in any decisions about their treatment (Bischoff et al. 2011, Courtenay et al. 2011, Vermeire et al. 2001). Hodder and Price (2009) suggest that patients should also be involved in the choice of inhaler device and this involvement will improve their adherence.

It is therefore important, when prescribing any new medication, that the patient is educated on its use and instructed on how to administer it. This education can affect any future adherence, including whether the patient even collects their first prescription (Lareau & Yawn 2010). In Tarn et *al.*'s (2006) study of 44 physicians issuing new prescriptions, fewer than 60% gave the patient full medication directions, such as the purpose of medication, the dosing quantity and frequency, or outlined the adverse effects. Some did not even mention the duration of treatment regimen. This certainly seems contrary to the Nursing and Midwifery Council's Standards of proficiency for nurse and midwife prescribers (NMC 2006).

Daily dosing versus more frequent regimes

Multiple dosing and/or inhaler use have been linked with higher rates of non-adherence in patients with COPD and it has been suggested that this is due to the increased complexity of having multiple dosing or devices (Mäkelä *et al.* 2013). Those patients who were initiated on once-daily dosing for their medication were found to have significantly higher adherence than those on other regimes (Toy *et al.* 2011); and Yu *et al.* (2011) showed that those patients who had to use their inhaler device multiple times did not persist with their treatment. The simple routine of a daily single long-acting inhaler has been shown to increase medication adherence in patients with both asthma and COPD (George *et al.* 2005).

Therapies that also combine medication within one inhaler have been shown to reduce moderate exacerbations, as in the TORCH study of **long-acting beta2 agonists** (**LABAs**) plus **inhaled corticosteroids** (**IHCs**) (Calverley *et al.* 2007). Wang *et al.* (2011) also showed that a combined regimen of the **long-acting muscarinic antagonist** (**LAMA**) tiotropium and a LABA (formoterol) reduced exacerbations. However, there is no confirmed link between the combination inhaler and reduced mortality (NICE 2012), as it is still unclear whether it is patient convenience that leads to greater treatment adherence or the action of the combined medication that reduces the exacerbations (Restrepo *et al.* 2008).

Education and medication beliefs

Medication beliefs are more powerful predictors of medical adherence than socio-demographic factors (Horne & Weinman 1999). A patient will consider their own beliefs about how important it is to have the medication and weigh it against their concerns about the potential side effects or adverse effects of taking their medication.

Self-management and action plans

Self-management that includes personal goals and health ambitions results in slower disease progression (Bourbeau *et al.* 2004). Patients themselves have highlighted their right to be treated in a holistic manner, whatever other health concerns they have. They have also requested that everyone involved in their care has the necessary skills, training and expertise (De Silva 2011). One way we can support our clients to self-manage their condition is to help them devise an action plan.

Read the following example.

Sample action plan

Personal details

Name:	Date of birth:	Doctor/Nurse:
Weight:	Height:	Best peak flow:

Medication (*Examples in italics*)

Reliever medication: *Salbutamol*	*2 puffs as required*	
Controller medication: *Qvar*	*1 puff bd*	
Green zone (This is best.)	**Amber zone** (My symptoms are getting worse.)	**Red zone** (I need help.)
Symptoms: • I have no **shortness of breath (SOB)** cough or chest discomfort. • I can do what I usually do. • I have no night-time symptoms.	Symptoms: • I'm coughing or wheezing or have chest tightness or SOB. • Symptoms keep me up at night. • I can do some things I usually do.	Symptoms: • I'm very short of breath. • I can't do my usual activities. • Quick-relief medicine doesn't help, or my symptoms are getting worse after 24 hours in the amber zone.
Peak flow: 80% or more of personal best.	Peak flow: 50–79% of personal best.	Peak flow: lower than 50% of personal best.
Action: Continue as usual.	Action: Medication: Take 2 puffs of salbutamol. Use a spacer device if I have one. If my symptoms don't get better or my peak flow has not returned to the green zone in 1 hour, then: Take 2 more puffs of salbutamol. If no improvement, move to red zone. If symptoms settle but night-time symptoms persist, double up preventer medication for 1 week. If symptoms persist, see Nurse/Doctor.	Action: Medication: Take 2 puffs of salbutamol. Repeat action if no improvement every 20 minutes until I feel relief or seek help. Double up Qvar. Begin prednisolone if I have a supply.
No further action.	Contact Nurse/Doctor if symptoms persist.	Contact Nurse/Doctor for urgent review.

Danger signs: Trouble walking and talking, due to shortness of breath. Lips or fingernails blue.

*Take 4 or 6 puffs of quick-relief medicine **and** seek urgent medical attention.*

Summary

Clearly, improving medical adherence will improve the patient's condition and will be more cost-effective for the NHS in general. There are strategies we can use, such as self-management and single-dose prescribing, that can improve adherence.

We have discussed why medical adherence is important for our patients. We know that it is defined by the World Health Organization (2003) as 'the extent to which a person's behaviour corresponds with the agreed recommendations from a healthcare provider'. We have also looked at why people do not take their prescribed medication and what strategies we can use to encourage them to do so. One effective method is to devise an action plan with our patients (as shown in the sample action plan included above).

Box 7.1b: Answers to reader activity

List five reasons why you think people do not take their medication as prescribed.

1. Cost of medication
2. Lack of knowledge
3. Concerns about side effects
4. Denial about their medical condition
5. Fear of what people think (stigmatisation).

References

Ágh, T., Inotai, A., Bártfai, Z. & Mészáros, Á. (2013). PRS-47 Relationship between medication adherence and quality of life in COPD–systematic review. *Value in Health.* **16**(7).

Ágh, T., Dömötör, P., Bártfai, Z., Inotai, A., Fujsz, E. & Mészáros, Á. (2014). Relationship between medication adherence and health-related quality of life in subjects with COPD: A systematic review. *Respiratory Care.* doi: 10.4187/respcare.03123.

Berger, B.E., Kapella, M.C. & Larson, J.L. (2010). The experience of stigma in chronic obstructive pulmonary disease. *Western Journal of Nursing Research.* doi:10.1177/0193945910384602

Bischoff, E.W., Hamd, D.H., Sedeno, M., Benedetti, A., Schermer, T.R., Bernard, S. & Bourbeau, J. (2011). Effects of written action plan adherence on COPD exacerbation recovery. *Thorax.* **66**(1), 26–31.

Bourbeau, J. & Bartlett, S.J. (2008). Patient adherence in COPD. *Thorax.* **63**(9), 831–838.

Bourbeau, J., Nault, D. & Dang-Tan, T. (2004). Self-management and behaviour modification in COPD. *Patient Education and Counseling.* **52**(3), 271–277.

Brown, M.T. & Bussell, J.K. (2011). Medication adherence: WHO cares? *Mayo Clinic Proceedings.* **86**, (4), 304–314.

Calverley, P.M., .A, Anderson, J.A. & Celli, B. (2007). Salmeterol and fluticasone propionate and survival in Chronic Obstructive Pulmonary Disease. *New England Journal of Medicine.* **356**, 775–789. http://www.nejm.org/doi/full/10.1056/NEJMoa063070 (Accessed 3.12.2016).

Challis, D., Hughes, J., Berzins, K. *et al.* (2010). Self-care and Case Management in Long-term Conditions: The effective management of critical interfaces. *National Institute for Health Research Service Delivery and Organisation Programme.* http://www.pssru.ac.uk/pdf/MCpdfs/SCCMfr.pdf (Accessed 3.12.2016).

Cochrane, G.M. (1992). Therapeutic compliance in asthma: its magnitude and implications. *European Respiratory Journal.* **5**, 122–124.

Courtenay, M., Carey, N., Stenner, K., Lawton, S. & Peters, J. (2011). Patients' views of nurse prescribing: effects on care, concordance and medicine taking. *British Journal of Dermatology.* **164**(2), 396–401.

Da Silva, D. (2011). Evidence: Helping people help themselves. A review of the evidence considering whether it is worthwhile to support self-management. *Health Foundation.* http://www.health.org.uk/sites/health/files/HelpingPeopleHelpThemselves.pdf (Accessed 3.12.2016).

DiMatteo, M.R., Giordani, P.J., Lepper, H.S. *et al.* (2002). Patient adherence and medical treatment outcomes: a meta-analysis. *Medical Care.* **40**, 794–011.

Dolce, J.J., Crisp, C., Manzella, B. *et al.* (1991). Medication adherence patterns in chronic obstructive pulmonary disease. *Chest.* **99**, 837–841.

Dompeling, E., Van Grunsven, P.M., Van Schayck, C.P. *et al.* (1992). Treatment with inhaled steroids in asthma and chronic bronchitis: long-term compliance and inhaler technique. *Family Practice.* **9**, 161–166.

Dowson, C.A., Town, G.I., Frampton, C. & Mulder, R.T. (2004). Psychopathology and illness beliefs influence COPD self-management. *Journal of Psychosomatic Research.* **56**, 333–340.

Egred, M., Shaw, S., Mohammad, B., Waitt, P. & Rodrigues, E. (2005). Under-use of beta-blockers in patients with ischaemic heart disease and concomitant chronic obstructive pulmonary disease. *QJM: An International Journal of Medicine.* **98**(7), 493–497.

George, J., Kong, D.C., Thoman, R. *et al.* (2005). Factors associated with medication nonadherence in patients with COPD. *Chest.* **128**, 3198–204.

George, J., Kong, D.C., Thoman, R. & Stewart, K. (2005). Factors associated with medication nonadherence in patients with COPD. *CHEST Journal.* **128**(5), 3198–3204.

George, J., Kong, D.C. & Stewart, K. (2007). Adherence to disease management programs in patients with COPD. *International Journal of Chronic Obstructive Pulmonary Disease.* **2**(3), 253.

Global Initiative for Chronic Obstructive Lung Disease (GOLD) (2016). *Global Strategy for Diagnosis, Management, and Prevention of COPD.* http://www.goldcopd.org/global-strategy-diagnosis-management-prevention-copd-2016/ (Accessed 3.12.2016).

Golay, A. (2011). Pharmacoeconomic aspects of poor adherence: can better adherence reduce healthcare costs? *Journal of Medical Economics.* **14**, 594–608

Hatton, M.Q., Allen, M.B., Vathenen, S.V. *et al.* (1996). Compliance with oral corticosteroids during steroid trials in chronic airways obstruction. *Thorax.* **51**, 323–324

Haynes, R.B., Taylor, D.W. & Sackett, D.L. (1979). *Compliance in Healthcare.* Baltimore, MD: Johns Hopkins University Press, pp. 1–7.

Hesselink, A.E., Penninx, B.W., Wijnhoven, H.A. *et al.* (2001). Determinants of an incorrect inhalation technique in patients with asthma or COPD. *Scandinavian Journal of Primary Health Care.* **19**, 255–60.

Hodder, R. & Price, D. (2009). Patient preferences for inhaler devices in chronic obstructive pulmonary disease: experience with Respimat® Soft Mist™ Inhaler. *International Journal of Chronic Obstructive Pulmonary Disease.* **4**, 381.

Horne, R. & Weinman, J. (1999). Patients' beliefs about prescribed medicines and their role in adherence to treatment in chronic physical illness. *Journal of Psychosomatic Research.* **47**(6), 555–567.

Johnson, J.L., Campbell, A.C., Bowers, M. & Nichol, A.M. (2007). Understanding the social consequences of chronic obstructive pulmonary disease: the effects of stigma and gender. *Proceedings of the American Thoracic Society.* **4**(8), 680–682.

Lareau, S.C. & Yawn, B.P. (2010). Improving adherence with inhaler therapy in COPD. *International Journal of Chronic Obstructive Pulmonary Disease.* **5**, 401.

Mäkelä, M.J., Backer, V., Hedegaard, M. & Larsson, K. (2013). Adherence to inhaled therapies, health outcomes and costs in patients with asthma and COPD. *Respiratory Medicine.* **107**(10), 1481–1490.

Mannino, D.M. & Braman, S. (2007). The epidemiology and economics of chronic obstructive pulmonary disease. *Proceedings of the American Thoracic Society.* **4**, 502–506.

Molimard, M. (2005). How to achieve good compliance and adherence with inhalation therapy. *Current Medical Research and Opinion®.* **21**(S4), S33–S37.

NICE (2012). *Chronic obstructive pulmonary disease. Evidence Update February 2012.* http://www.nice.org.uk/guidance/cg101/evidence/cg101-chronic-obstructive-pulmonary-disease-updated-evidence-update2 (Accessed 3.12.2016).

Nursing & Midwifery Council (NMC) (2006). *Standards of proficiency for nurse and midwife prescribers.* http://www.nmc-uk.org/Documents/NMC-Publications/NMC-Standards-proficiency-nurse-and-midwife-prescribers.pdf (Accessed 3.12.2016).

Partridge, M.R. (2004). Living with COPD: the patients' perspective. *European Respiratory Review.* **13**(88), 1–5.

Pauwels, R.A., Buist, A.S., Calverley, P.M. *et al.* (2001). Global strategy for the diagnosis, management, and prevention of chronic obstructive pulmonary disease. NHLBI/WHO Global Initiative for Chronic Obstructive Lung Disease (GOLD) Workshop summary. *American Journal of Respiratory and Critical Care Medicine.* **163**, 1256–1276.

Pepin, J.L., Barjhoux, C.E., Deschaux, C. *et al.* (1996). Long-term oxygen therapy at home. Compliance with medical prescription and effective use of therapy. ANTADIR Working Group on Oxygen Therapy. Association Nationale de Traitement a Domicile des Insuffisants Respiratoires. *Chest.* **109**, 1144–1150.

Piette, J.D., Heisler, M. & Wagner, T.H. (2004). Cost-related medication underuse among chronically ill adults: the treatments people forgo, how often, and who is at risk. *American Journal of Public Health.* **94**(10), 1782–1787.

Purdy, S., Paranjothy, S., Huntley, A. *et al.* (2012). Interventions to reduce unplanned hospital admission: a series of systematic reviews, National Institute for Health Research/University of Bristol. http://www.bristol.ac.uk/primaryhealthcare/docs/projects/unplannedadmissions.pdf (Accessed 3.12.2016).

Ramsey, S.D. (2000). Suboptimal medical therapy in COPD: exploring the causes and consequences. *Chest.* **117**: 33S–37S.

Rand, C.S. (2005). Patient adherence with COPD therapy. *European Respiratory Review.* **14**, 97–101.

Restrepo, R.D., Alvarez, M.T., Wittnebel, L.D., Sorenson, H., Wettstein, R., Vines, D.L. & Wilkins, R.L. (2008). Medication adherence issues in patients treated for COPD. *International Journal of Chronic Obstructive Pulmonary Disease.* **3**(3), 371.

Rice, K.L., Dewan, N., Bloomfield, H.E. *et al.* (2010) Disease management program for chronic obstructive pulmonary disease: a randomized controlled trial. *American Journal of Respiratory and Critical Care Medicine.* **182**, 890–896. https://www.ncbi.nlm.nih.gov/pubmed/20075385 (Accessed 3.12.2016).

Tarn, D.M., Heritage, J., Paterniti, D.A., Hays, R.D., Kravitz, R.L. & Wenger, N.S. (2006). Physician communication when prescribing new medications. *Archives of Internal Medicine.* **166**, 1855–1862.

The Global Initiative for Asthma (GINA) (2016). *The pocket guide for asthma management and prevention.* http://ginasthma.org/2016-pocket-guide-for-asthma-management-and-prevention/ (Accessed 3.12.2016).

Toy, E.L., Beaulieu, N.U., McHale, J.M., Welland, T.R., Plauschinat, C.A., Swensen, A. & Duh, M.S. (2011). Treatment of COPD: relationships between daily dosing frequency, adherence, resource use, and costs. *Respiratory Medicine.* **105**(3), 435–441.

Turner, J., Wright, E., Mendella, L. & Anthonisen, N. (1995). Predictors of patient adherence to long-term home nebulizer therapy for COPD. *CHEST Journal.* **108**(2), 394–400.

van Boven, J.F., Chavannes, N.H., van der Molen, T., Rutten-van Mölken, M.P., Postma, M.J. & Vegter, S. (2014). Clinical and economic impact of non-adherence in COPD: a systematic review. *Respiratory Medicine.* **108**(1), 103–113.

Vermeire, E., Hearnshaw, H., Van Royen, P., & Denekens, J. (2001). Patient adherence to treatment: three decades of research. A comprehensive review. *Journal of Clinical Pharmacy and Therapeutics.* **26**(5), 331–342.

Yu, A., Guerin, D., Ponce de Leon, K., Ramakrishnan, E.Q., Wu, M. *et al.* (2011). Therapy persistence and adherence in patients with chronic obstructive pulmonary disease: multiple versus single long-acting maintenance inhalers. *Journal of Medical Economics.* **14**, 486–496

Walters, J.A.E., Turnock, A.C., Walters, E.H. *et al.* (2010). Action plans with limited patient education only for exacerbations of chronic obstructive pulmonary disease. *Cochrane Database of Systematic Reviews.* Issue 5: CD005074. www.onlinelibrary.wiley.com/doi/10.1002/14651858.CD005074.pub3/pdf (Accessed 3.12.2016).

Wang, J., Jin, D., Zuo, P. *et al.* (2011) Comparison of tiotropium plus formoterol to tiotropium alone in stable chronic obstructive pulmonary disease: a meta-analysis. *Respirology.* **16**, 350–8 http://www.onlinelibrary.wiley.com/doi/10.1111/j.1440-1843.2010.01912.x/abstract (Accessed 3.12.2016).

World Health Organization (WHO) (2003). *Adherence to long-term therapies: evidence for action.* http://www.who.int/chp/knowledge/publications/adherence_report/en/ (Accessed 3.12.2016).

World Health Organization (WHO) (November 2016). *Chronic Obstructive Pulmonary Disease (COPD) Fact Sheet No 315.* http://www.who.int/mediacentre/factsheets/fs315/en/index.html (Accessed 3.12.2016).

Chapter 8

Pharmacology

In this chapter, we will look at the look at the main categories of medication prescribed for patients with respiratory disease, such as bronchodilators, antihistamines and antibiotics. We will also review some of the new surgical options that are available when managing obstructive respiratory conditions.

Commonly used medication in respiratory disease

There are five main types of inhaled medication that are used for respiratory disease and these are generally delivered using an inhaler device. This section will also provide a short summary of the other drugs that are used.

Box 8.1: Inhaled drugs commonly used in respiratory disease

- Short-acting beta2 agonists (SABAs)
- Short-acting muscarinic antagonists (SAMAs)
- Long-acting beta agonists (LABAs) or once-daily LABA
- Long-acting muscarinic antagonists (LAMAs)
- Inhaled corticosteriods (IHCs)

Bronchodilator sympathomimetics stimulate the beta2-receptors, causing the level of cellular cAMP to increase. The airway smooth muscles relax, creating bronchodilation.

Short-acting beta2 agonists

SABAs are called 'rescue' medication, as they work within 2–3 minutes of inhalation and are prescribed for the short-term relief of breathlessness. Certainly, for patients experiencing an acute exacerbation of COPD, short-acting inhaled beta2 agonists are the preferred bronchodilators (GOLD 2016, NICE 2010). They are quick-acting medications but only have a short duration of 3–4 hours. Examples are fenoterol, salbutamol and terbutaline.

Side effects of SABAs

Approximately 10% of patients can experience adverse reactions to the medication they are prescribed. These reactions vary depending on the amount of medication that has been inhaled or absorbed. The most common reactions that occur with SABAs are:

- Unpleasant and unusual taste
- Mouth and throat irritation
- Fine tremor (usually the hands)
- Nausea, sweating, restlessness
- Headache and dizziness
- Paradoxical bronchospasm with inhaled therapies.

Beta2 agonists also stimulate beta1 receptors, which leads to side effects such as **tachycardia**. These are more common when the medication is ingested or the patient is inhaling large amounts of their medication. Other side effects may include:

- Paroxysmal **tachyarrhythmias**, such as **atrial fibrillation** or paroxysmal supraventricular tachycardia
- Tremors
- Headaches
- Hyperactive behaviour, particularly in children
- Muscle cramps
- Insomnia
- A general feeling of anxiety and nervousness
- In high doses, beta2 agonists can cause hypokalaemia and hyperglycaemia.

Box 8.2a: Reader activity

List the five main types of inhaled medication used in respiratory disease.

Long-acting beta agonists

Unlike short-acting beta agonists, LABAs are prescribed to aid control of symptoms (rather than immediate relief) and are classified as maintenance medications. They can aid bronchodilation for up to 12 hours or more. New forms of this medication are being trialled with a longer half-life, a once-a-day profile and to be combined with IHCs (Lötvall *et al.* 2012).

The most common types of LABA are formoterol (Oxis, Foradil) and salmeterol (Serevent). Formoterol is quick acting (reaching its peak at 4−6 hours) and can remain in the bloodstream for up to 12 hours. Salmeterol works within 20 minutes and lasts 12 hours (Lötvall 2001).

Not only do these drugs help to control symptoms but they also enhance the anti-inflammatory action of corticosteroids and can be delivered in combination with IHCs. Despite the significant benefits of these drugs for patients with **asthma** and COPD, there has been widespread debate about their safety. This is because LABAs may cause adverse cardiovascular effects, such as hypokalaemia, heart palpitations and ventricular arrhythmias, as they are beta2-adrenoceptor agonists, which are also found in cardiac tissue (Rossi et al. 2008). In 2004 the results were published from a large three-year prospective randomised trial (TORCH study) comparing the effects of salmeterol with a placebo (Vestbo 2004). The patients who had been prescribed salmeterol had better quality of life scores, lung function results and lower levels of mortality (Rossi et al. 2008, Vestbo 2004). The recommendations of the TORCH study were therefore incorporated in the 2004 British Thoracic Society guidelines, which were updated in 2014 (BTS 2014).

Muscarinic antagonists

SAMAs are also bronchodilators. Examples of short-acting muscarinics are ipratropium or atrovent, which block the muscarinic effects of acetylcholine. However, ipratropium bromide has been associated with an increased risk of adverse cardiovascular effects and acute angle-closure glaucoma (Ogale et al. 2010).

LAMAs have been shown to offer significant improvements for patients with COPD in their lung function, easing their symptoms and improving their quality of life (Braido et al. 2013, Yohannes et al. 2011). They have been shown to reduce the number of exacerbations a patient has in a year (Braido et al. 2013) and have also been shown to improve the lung function of patients with small airways disease and **cystic fibrosis** (Kerstjens et al. 2012, Zeitlin 2007). Patients with poorly controlled asthma found that adding tiotropium to their IHCs and LAMAs significantly increased the time before their first severe exacerbation and provided sustained bronchodilation (Kerstjens et al. 2012).

The most common type of LAMA is tiotropium. Other examples include: glycopyrronium, aclidinium and umeclidinium.

Cautions regarding LAMAs

Any patient who has had a myocardial infarction in the past 6 months, or who is unstable or has life-threatening cardiac arrhythmia or has been hospitalised for heart failure in the past year, is at high risk of experiencing further cardiovascular events if they are prescribed LAMAs and should be regularly reviewed (BNF 2016b).

Side effects of LAMAs

Side effects range from **dysphonia**, taste disorders, gastrointestinal disorders and **candida** of the **oropharynx** to muscle pain and dry mouth. Patients may also experience joint swelling and sleep disturbances (BNF 2016b).

Inhaled corticosteroids

IHCs have been shown to be effective in patients with asthma, as they reduce airway hyper-responsiveness, inhibit the migration and activation of inflammatory cells and block late phase reaction to **allergens**. They also promote the action of beta-adrenergic receptor activity. In general, IHCs are well tolerated and safe at the recommended dosages.

The efficacy and side effects of IHCs depend on the dose and type of corticosteroid. However, for people with COPD, the evidence is unclear so they are not used as a first-line treatment in this patient group (GOLD 2016).

Side effects of IHCs

The main side effects of inhaled corticosteroids occur because the drug is deposited into the oropharynx and larynx. Dysphonia (a hoarse voice) is a common side effect as well as candida. These oropharyngeal disorders are the most common side effects of IHCs, which is also the main reason why patients with asthma or COPD have poor adherence to the drug (Molimard et al. 2010).

Cromolyn

Cromolyn is a mast cell stabiliser which prevents mast cells releasing histamine. This drug is delivered by aerosol and inhaled by the patient. However, leukotriene receptor antagonists have more or less replaced the use of cromolyn.

Phosphodiesterase-4 inhibitor

Phosphodiesterase-4 is a member of the PDE enzyme, which is involved in preventing cyclic adenosine monophosphate and cyclic guanosine monophosphate.

The once-daily phosphodiesterase-4 inhibitor, roflumilast, targets the inflammatory processes underlying COPD and therefore reduces the number of exacerbations these patients experience. It is effective for patients with severe air flow limitation and frequent exacerbations that are not adequately controlled by long-acting bronchodilators (GOLD 2016).

Side effects of phosphodiesterase-4 inhibitors

The main side effects are nausea, vomiting, diarrhoea, headaches and weight loss. There is also a risk of mental illness. In general, phosphodiesterase-4 inhibitors, such as roflumilast, are considered to be safe and effective for the treatment of COPD (Lipari & Kale-Pradhan 2014).

Mucolytics

Mucolytics are prescribed to patients with COPD to facilitate expectoration by reducing **sputum** viscosity. It has a mucoregulation effect, causing the mucus to become less viscous and aiding its clearance from the respiratory tract (BNF 2016a). It also has beneficial effects in patients who suffer from frequent exacerbations. For over ten years, research has shown that the use of mucolytics is linked with a reduction in the number of acute exacerbations a patient can experience and the number of days in hospital (Poole & Black 2001, Gerrits *et al.* 2003). In a study of patients after one year of treatment with high-dose N-acetylcysteine, Tse *et al.* (2013) found that there was a significant improvement, involving less frequent exacerbations and enhanced small airway function.

Leukotriene receptor antagonists

Leukotriene receptor antagonists work in the airways to block the effects of cysteinyl leukotrienes, which are usually released by the mast cells, **basophils** and **eosinophils**. If the leukotrienes are released, they cause airway constriction, an increase in mucus production, and swelling and inflammation in the lungs. The two commonly prescribed drugs for this condition are montelukast and zafirlukast, which are thought to help ease exercise-induced asthma and reduce symptoms in those with allergic **rhinitis**.

Side effects of leukotriene receptor antagonists

Commonly occurring side effects include: abdominal pain, thirst, headache, and **hyperkinesia** (in young children). Less common side effects are: dry mouth, **dyspepsia**, **oedema**, dizziness, drowsiness, malaise, sleep disturbances, abnormal dreams, anxiety, agitation, depression, psychomotor hyperactivity, **paraesthesia**, **hypoesthesia**, seizures, **arthralgia**, **myalgia** and **epistaxis**. **Churg-Strauss syndrome** is rare but has occurred with the use of leukotriene receptor antagonists.

Oral bronchodilators

Methylxanthines, such as theophylline and aminophylline, are oral bronchodilators. Xanthines are thought to relax the smooth muscle in the airway and increase diaphragm contractility. They are nonselective phosphodiesterase inhibitors, which have a moderately potent bronchodilator action that is similar to caffeine. Patients starting the medication should have their serum levels checked within 5 days of starting it. They also need to remain on the same modified-release form of methylxanthine, as the absorption rates vary from brand to brand. Other factors, such as age, gender and smoking, may also affect absorption rates (Khan *et al.* 2014).

Aminophylline should be reserved for severe acute asthma that fails to respond to standard management, particularly in an intravenous form (British Thoracic Society 2014). Theophylline should be considered for patients who do not get relief from standard bronchodilators (see Figure 6.2: Stepwise asthma management, p. 71). The oral form of this medication is in a modified-release format, which has had the timing and/or rate of release of the drug substance altered. This enables a slow, steady release of the medication, without peaks and troughs of absorption. The rate of absorption of these preparations can also vary from brand to brand. The patient should therefore remain on the same branded medication while they are prescribed the drug.

IHCs are contraindicated for women who are pregnant or breastfeeding. If patients are stable on their medication, the medication should not be changed.

Side effects of oral bronchodilators

These drugs do have several unpleasant side effects, including:

- Nausea and vomiting

- Insomnia

- Cardiac arrhythmias

- Seizures

- Hypokalaemia.

It is also important to remember that the liver enzymes responsible for theophylline metabolism do not work effectively when taken with the following types of antibiotics: macrolides such as erythromycin and quinolones such as ciprofloxacin. Patients should also have their liver function reviewed on a regular basis.

Cholinesterase inhibitors

These drugs include bambuterol, which is another long-acting beta adrenoceptor agonist (LABA) prescribed for the management of asthma, bronchospasm and/or reversible airways obstruction (eMC 2016).

Cholinesterase inhibitor contraindications and cautions

This drug is contraindicated in people with severe liver impairment, impaired renal function and pregnancy. Caution should be taken and patients carefully observed if they have thyrotoxicosis, as with other beta2 agonists.

Possible side effects include:

- Tachycardia

- Arrhythmias

- Raised blood sugar levels

- Hypokalaemia.

Antihistamines

Antihistamines are used for patients with allergic asthma, as they block the work of histamine which is one of the chemical mediators of inflammation. There are first-generation antihistamines that have more anticholinergic side effects, such as drowsiness and a dry mouth. The second-generation antihistamines have few side effects, and these drugs are commonly used for allergic rhinitis and allergic **sinusitis**.

Caution should be exercised when prescribing antihistamines for those with kidney and liver problems; and these drugs should not be prescribed for pregnant women or patients with prolonged QT waves.

Antibiotics

With a growing increase in antimicrobial resistance, it is important to ensure that your patient is prescribed the appropriate antibiotics, *only* when they are needed, and that the treatment is selected based on local guidelines. Suggestions also include using the recommended dose with the narrowest spectrum of activity, the fewest side effects and at the lowest cost. The most common type of antibiotic prescribed for lower respiratory infections, such as bronchitis, is amoxicillin. However, there is some debate regarding the effectiveness of amoxicillin as antibiotic therapy – especially in older patients (Little *et al.* 2012).

Amoxicillin is a beta-lactam antibiotic like penicillin and is commonly used to treat bacterial infections caused by susceptible microorganisms. It is also appropriate for uncomplicated bacterial rhinosinusitis, **otitis media**, sinusitis, and infections caused by susceptible organisms involving the upper and lower respiratory tract, particularly group A streptococcal infections.

Cephalosporins are a group of broad-spectrum, semi-synthetic beta-lactam antibiotics. They originated from the mould Cephalosporium – hence the name. They are similar to penicillins in action, as they damage the bacterial cell wall synthesis. Cefaclor is a second-generation cephalosporin that works on gram-positive bacteria such as P mirabilis, H influenzae, E coli, Klebsiella pneumoniae and Moraxella catarrhalis. The other medication that is commonly used is Cefuroxime, which is a second-generation cephalosporin and can be used against P mirabilis, H influenzae, E coli, K pneumoniae and M catarrhalis.

Macrolides block the cells' protein synthesis. They are used for the treatment of group A streptococcal infection in patients with penicillin sensitivity. They can also be used for rhinosinusitis, **pertussis** and **diphtheria**. Erythromycin is the commonest macrolide for penicillin allergies. It is also effective for rhinosinusitis, staphylococcal and streptococcal infections. Azithromycin is another macrolide commonly used for upper and lower respiratory tract infections.

Antibiotics are considered the mainstay for most respiratory infections, although most upper respiratory infections are caused by viral infections and will resolve spontaneously without prescribed medication. It is therefore important to recognise bacterial infections and assess which is the appropriate antibiotic to use to treat it. It is also important to adhere to national and local prescribing guidelines, as resistance can vary from one area to another.

Nebuliser therapy

Nebuliser therapy converts liquid into aerosol droplets, which can be inhaled. It is therefore a suitable delivery system for patients with respiratory disease, as the droplets are easier to inhale and the drug is delivered straight to the site of action (Rees 2005). However, it is no more effective than using a metered-dose inhaler delivered by spacer in adults or children (Cates *et al.* 2013). There are also effective ways to ensure children receive the correct dosage of their medication via a space device such as a whistling mask. It is an effective delivery system for aqueous vapour, which is used for patients with COPD who have copious amounts of mucus.

The nebuliser is thought to reduce the viscosity of mucus and help the patient with expectoration. The use of high oxygen flow regulators with nebulisers is also recommended in the British Thoracic Society guidelines (BTS 2014) for life-threatening asthma.

Long-term inhaled antibiotic therapy has been used to treat **bronchiectasis** and cystic fibrosis for several years (Hodson *et al.* 2002, Mukhopadhyay *et al.* 1996, Orriols *et al.* 1999). It has therefore been shown to be an effective way of delivering antibiotics for patients with these long-term conditions.

Nebulisers may also be considered for the delivery of corticosteroids (such as budesonide), as the medication is delivered to the site of inflammation. This may be an effective alternative to systemic corticosteroids, especially in conditions such as COPD (Gunen *et al.* 2007).

Immunisation

Immunisation is another tool in the care of a patient with respiratory disease. The main vaccinations used to prevent respiratory disease are: seasonal and pandemic influenza vaccinations, pertussis, pneumococcal disease and **tuberculosis**.

Bordetella pertussis (whooping cough) can lead to 300,000 deaths each year in the immunosuppressed groups such as babies and children, despite being the leading vaccine-preventable cause of death (ERS 2016). It can also lead to complications or exacerbations in patients with other long-term diseases such as COPD. The PPV-23 pneumococcal vaccine also prevents these complications in those in the at-risk groups.

There is some debate about whether the influenza vaccination might aggravate respiratory symptoms but the benefit of the vaccine outweighs the risk of symptoms and it is certainly recommended for a number of chronic respiratory diseases (BTS 2014, GOLD 2016, Nicholson *et al.* 1998).

Surgery

There have been several developments in respiratory surgery over the last decade. Some of the more successful options are outlined below:

Lung volume reduction surgery

Lung volume reduction surgery (LVRS), used to resect areas that have emphysemic changes in COPD, has been shown to improve outcomes for selected patient groups (Criner 2011). Bronchoscopic lung volume reduction (BLVR) that allows air to leave but not enter emphysematous areas of the lung is not yet recommended outside clinical trials (GOLD 2016, Davey *et al.* 2015).

Bronchial thermaplasty

Bronchial thermaplasty (BT) can be used to reduce the mass of smooth muscle in the walls of conducting airways. This is often thickened due to scarring. This in turn reduces the potential for smooth muscle-mediated bronchoconstriction. This procedure has been found to be well tolerated in patients with asthma. Patients have been found to have a decrease in their airway hyper-responsiveness and this improvement can last for at least two years (Cox *et al.* 2006). It is still only available in specialist centres, for those with difficult-to-manage asthma (NICE 2012). There also needs to be further research into any potential long-term effects (such as stenosis) due to this treatment.

Summary

There are various pharmacological options for patients with respiratory disease, a number of which are outlined in this chapter. As researchers look at the mechanisms involved in respiratory disease, the hope is that new pharmacological developments will emerge. One example is the work of Kume (2016) who has looked at the synergistic effects between beta2 adrenergic receptors and the muscarinic receptors. A novel approach to bronchodilator therapy would be to include drugs that act on both pathways. There are already new combination drugs such as Stiolto Respimat, which contains tiotropium and olodaterol, which are effective as long-acting bronchiodilators (eMC 2016). Another innovative treatment is the regeneration of damaged alveoli and this is still at an early experimental stage (Todd *et al.* 2014).

Box 8.2b: Answers to reader activity

List the five main types of inhaled medication used in respiratory disease.

1. Short-acting beta agonists (SABAs)
2. Short-acting muscarinic antagonists (SAMAs)
3. Long-acting beta agonists (LABAs)
4. Long-acting muscarinic antagonists (LAMAs)
5. Inhaled corticosteroids (IHCs)

References

BNF (2016a). *Mucolytics.*
http://www.evidence.nhs.uk/formulary/bnf/current/3-respiratory-system/37-mucolytics (Accessed 5.12.2016).

BNF (2016b). https://www.evidence.nhs.uk/formulary/bnf/current/3-respiratory-system/31-bronchodilators/312-antimuscarinic-bronchodilators/tiotropium (Accessed 5.12.2016).

Braido, F., Baiardini, I., Cazzola, M., Brusselle, G., Marugo, F. & Canonica, G. (2013). Long acting bronchodilators improve health related quality of life in patients with COPD. *Respiratory Medicine.* **107**, 1465–1480.

British Thoracic Society (2014). SIGN 141. *British guideline on the management of asthma.* https://www.brit-thoracic.org.uk/document-library/clinical-information/asthma/btssign-asthma-guideline-2014 (Accessed 5.12.2016).

Cates, C.J., Welsh, E. & Rowe, B.H. (2013). Holding chambers (spacers) versus nebulisers for beta-agonist treatment of acute asthma. *Cochrane Database of Systematic Reviews.* **13**, 9.

Cox, G., Miller, J.D., McWilliams, A., FitzGerald, J.M. & Lam, S. (2006). Bronchial thermoplasty for asthma. *American Journal of Respiratory and Critical Care Medicine.* **173**(9), 965–969.

Criner, G. (2011). Lung volume reduction as an alternative to transplantation for COPD. *Clinical Chest Medicine.* **32**(2), 379–397.

Davey, C., Zoumot, Z., Jordan, S., Carr, D., Polkey, M., Shah, P. & Hopkinson, N. (2015). Bronchoscopic lung volume reduction with endobronchial valves for patients with heterogeneous emphysema and intact interlobar fissures (The BeLieVeR-HIFi trial): study design and rationale. *Thorax.* **70**, 288–290.

electronic Medicines Compendium (eMC) (2016). Bambec. https://www.medicines.org.uk/emc/medicine/9574 (Accessed 5.12.2016).

European Respiratory Society (ERS) (2016). *European Lung White Book.* http://www.erswhitebook.org/chapters/immunisation-against-respiratory-diseases/ (Accessed 5.12.2016).

Gerrits, C.M.J.M., Herings, R.M.C., Leufkens, H.G.M., & Lammers, J.J. (2003). N-acetylcysteine reduces the risk of re-hospitalisation among patients with chronic obstructive pulmonary disease. *European Respiratory Journal.* **21**(5), 795–798.

Global Initiative for Chronic Obstructive Lung Disease (GOLD) (2016). *Global Strategy for Diagnosis, Management, and Prevention of COPD.* http://www.goldcopd.org/global-strategy-diagnosis-management-prevention-copd-2016/ (Accessed 3.12.2016).

Gunen, H., Hacievliyagil, S.S., Yetkin, O., Gulbas, G., Mutlu, L.C., & In, E. (2007). The role of nebulised budesonide in the treatment of exacerbations of COPD. *European Respiratory Journal.* **29**(4), 660–667

Hodson, M.E., Gallagher, C.G., & Govan, J.R.W. (2002). A randomised clinical trial of nebulised tobramycin or colistin in cystic fibrosis. *European Respiratory Journal.* **20**(3), 658–664.

Kume, H. (2016). *Towards a cure for asthma and pulmonary disease. International Innovation.* http://www.internationalinnovation.com/towards-cure-asthma-pulmonary-disease/ (Accessed 12.12.2016).

Kerstjens, H.A., Engel, M., Dahl, R., Paggiaro, P., Beck, E., Vandewalker, M. & Bateman, E.D. (2012). Tiotropium in asthma poorly controlled with standard combination therapy. *New England Journal of Medicine.* **367**(13), 1198–1207.

Khan, S., Jones, S. & Preston, C. (2014). Theophylline. *The Pharmaceutical Journal.* 293(7818) online. DOI: 10.1211/PJ.2014.20065570 http://www.pharmaceutical-journal.com/learning/learning-article/theophylline-interactions/20065570.article#fn_6 (Accessed 5.12.2016).

Little, P., Stuart, B., Moore, M. et al. (2012). Amoxicillin for acute lower-respiratory-tract infection in primary care when pneumonia is not suspected: a 12-country, randomised, placebo-controlled trial. *The Lancet Infectious Diseases.* DOI: http://dx.doi.org/10.1016/S1473-3099(12)70300-6 (Accessed 5.12.2016).

Lipari, M. & Kale-Pradhan, P.B. (2014). Vulnerable COPD patients with comorbidities: the role of roflumilast. *Journal of Therapeutics & Clinical Risk Management.* **18** (10), 969–976.

Lötvall, J. (2001). Pharmacological similarities and differences between β2-agonists. *Respiratory Medicine.* **95**, S7–S11.

Lötvall, J., Bateman, E.D., Bleecker, E.R., Busse, W.W., Woodcock, A., Follows, R. & Haumann, B. (2012). 24-h duration of the novel LABA vilanterol trifenatate in asthma patients treated with inhaled corticosteroids. *European Respiratory Journal.* **40**(3), 570–579.

Molimard, M., Gros, V.L., Robinson, P. & Bourdeix, I. (2010). Prevalence and associated factors of oropharyngeal side effects in users of inhaled corticosteroids in a real-life setting. *Journal of Aerosol Medicine and Pulmonary Drug Delivery.* **23**(2), 91–95.

Mukhopadhyay, S., Singh, M., Cater, J.I., Ogston, S., Franklin, M. & Olver, R.E. (1996). Nebulised antipseudomonal antibiotic therapy in cystic fibrosis: a meta-analysis of benefits and risks. *Thorax.* **51**(4), 364–368.

National Institute for Clinical Excellence (NICE). (2010). *Chronic obstructive pulmonary disease in over 16s: diagnosis and management.* https://www.nice.org.uk/guidance/CG101 (Accessed 5.12.2016).

National Institute for Clinical Excellence (NICE). (2012). *Bronchial thermoplasty for severe asthma.* https://www.nice.org.uk/guidance/ipg419 (Accessed 5.12.2016).

Nicholson, K.G., Nguyen-Van-Tam, J.S., Ahmed, A.H., Wiselka, M.J., Leese, J., Ayres, J. *et al.* (1998). Randomised placebo-controlled crossover trial on effect of inactivated influenza vaccine on pulmonary function in asthma. *Lancet.* **351**(9099), 326–331.

Ogale, S., Lee, T., Boudreau, D. & Sullivan, S.D. (2010) Cardiovascular events associated with ipratropium bromide in COPD. *Chest.* **137**, 13–19.

Orriols, R., Roig, J., Ferrer, J., Sampol, G., Rosell, A., Ferrer, A. & Vallano, A. (1999). Inhaled antibiotic therapy in non-cystic fibrosis patients with bronchiectasis and chronic bronchial infection by Pseudomonas aeruginosa. *Respiratory Medicine.* **93**(7), 476–480.

Poole, P.J. & Black, P.N. (2001). Oral mucolytic drugs for exacerbations of chronic obstructive pulmonary disease: systematic review. *British Medical Journal.* **322**(7297), 1271.

Rees, J. (2005). Methods of delivering drugs. *British Medical Journal.* **331**(7515), 504–506.

Rossi, A., Khirani, S. & Cazzola, M. (2008). Long-acting β2-agonists (LABA) in chronic obstructive pulmonary disease: efficacy and safety. *International Journal of Chronic Obstructive Pulmonary Disease.* **4**, 521–529.

Tse, H.N., Raiteri, L., Wong, K.Y., Yee, K.S., Ng, L.Y., Wai, K.Y. & Chan, M.H. (2013). High-dose N-acetylcysteine in stable COPD: the 1-year, double-blind, randomized, placebo-controlled HIACE study. *CHEST Journal.* **144**(1), 106–118.

Todd, J.L., Jain, R., Pavlisko, E N., Finlen Copeland, C.A., Reynolds, J.M., Snyder, L.D., & Palmer, S.M. (2014). Impact of forced vital capacity loss on survival after the onset of chronic lung allograft dysfunction. *American Journal of Respiratory and Critical Care Medicine.* **189**(2), 159–166.

Vestbo, J. (2004). The TORCH (towards a revolution in COPD health) survival study protocol. TORCH Study Group. *European Respiratory Journal.* **24**(2), 206–210.

Yohannes, A., Willgoss, T. & Vestbo, J. (2011). Tiotropium for the treatment of stable COPD: a meta-analysis of clinically relevant outcomes. *Respiratory Care.* **56**, 477–487.

Zeitlin, P.L. (2007). Emerging drug treatments for cystic fibrosis. *Expert Opinion on Emerging Drugs.* **12**(2), 329–336.

Chapter 9

Intermediate, home-based and end of life care

Patients with respiratory disease often have someone who helps them with their personal, emotional or practical care. This is usually an unpaid role and may be delivered by a family member or a friend. They can manage this form of care if they are supported by the patient's doctor and local social services, with intermittent help from secondary healthcare services and sometimes third sector involvement.

However, the patient may reach a stage where they need more care than their families or friends can provide. This can be a frightening time, when they may experience increasing breathlessness or have to cope with more frequent exacerbations. They may want to remain at home and won't necessarily want to go to hospital. These patients often have complex care needs and need the additional support of community and hospital services.

Intermediate care

Intermediate care is a model of treatment that sits at the interface between hospital and the community setting. It means being cared for 'in between' services or a seamless continuum of care between services (DH 2001). It was initially an alternative to hospital admission and care for elderly patients in the *NHS plan* (DH 2004). It has been found to be an effective service for patients with a chronic respiratory disease, such as **chronic obstructive pulmonary disorder (COPD)**, with frequent exacerbations. Prior to the establishment of the intermediate care service, such patients had a high level of hospital inpatient stays.

The main aim of intermediate care is to support and empower patients, to encourage independence and the prevention of unnecessary admission to hospital (Melis *et al.* 2004). This is similar to the Audit Commission's (2000) definition of intermediate care, which states that the 'primary function of intermediate care is to build up people's confidence to cope once more with day-to-day activities'.

It involves collaborative care between all the health professionals who care for the patient, including, for example, GPs, social workers, dieticians, physiotherapists, specialist nurses and community pharmacists.

Each patient in intermediate care will expect to have:

- An individual plan of care that includes a review of their health and social care
- Regular monitoring
- A review of the services they receive
- A person-centred programme of rehabilitation involving a multidisciplinary team
- A continuation of such programmes after they have been discharged from a clinical setting.

One example of a nurse-led intermediate care package for patients with COPD includes pulmonary rehabilitation, self- management education, personalised action plans, frequent telephone reviews and visits by a specialist nurse, although these can vary from service to service (Sridhar et al. 2008). Although this service has been shown to reduce acute use of primary care services and lead to a reduction in patient mortality, it has not been associated with a decrease in acute admission rates to secondary care (Sridhar et al. 2008). Other forms of intermediate care delivery have been developed such as asthma and COPD day care units.

Home-based care

A client who is receiving home care is based in their home, with their social network around them, but receives home carers as part of the intermediate care team. These patients will be given a thorough health and social assessment and their plan will include goals and regular reviews (Kent et al. 2002).

Patients with COPD may find home-based care particularly beneficial. It is considered to be a safe and effective treatment approach for certain patients with exacerbations of COPD (Oliveira et al. 2011). Certainly, there were found to be no significant differences for patients with COPD who were in hospital or using home-based care. This was assessed using FEV1, readmission rates, mortality and the number of days in care (Davies et al. 2000, Skwarska et al. 2000). Ram et al. (2004) did find that home-based care was less expensive than inpatient care.

We want to focus on what patients themselves think about the service, as patient satisfaction is an important component of care quality. Davison et al. (2012) suggest their study of home-based care supported early discharge of patients with COPD and more appropriate use of the acute services. Patients had received self-management education and knew when it was appropriate to seek medical help. Meanwhile, Richards et al. (1998) showed that patients receiving home-based care had higher levels of perceived involvement in the decision-making processes.

Provision of good-quality end of life care is also something we need to plan for, as the percentage of people living into old age with serious respiratory conditions is increasing rapidly. Patient-centred care should involve meeting these patients' needs in a timely manner, rather than responding to a diagnosis (Addington-Hall 1998).

End of life care

Patients with end-stage COPD or other respiratory disease usually have a significantly impaired quality of life and reduced emotional well-being. Despite the high mortality and morbidity rates associated with this degenerative condition, these patients often receive poor palliative care. They have found that their needs have often not been met as effectively as patients with lung cancer (Gore et al. 2010, Curtis 2008).

The two major factors that may influence the quality of end of life care are the presence of anxiety and depression associated with this long-term condition and the lack of advance care planning (Curtis 2008). Perhaps the disparity between end of life care for lung cancer sufferers and those with other respiratory diseases is partly due to the difficulty in identifying when the patient has reached the end of life stage. Certainly, those with long-term respiratory illness, who are managed outside cancer services, are often overlooked. In addition, the patient's deteriorating health status, decreased independence, social isolation and family stresses due to the disease often mean they don't seek help when they need it (Fitzsimmons et al. 2007). There is also a lack of resources available to the teams caring for these patients, as so many resources are focused on the acutely ill patient (Skilbeck et al. 1998). There therefore needs to be an earlier and more effective implementation of the palliative care approach if the needs of patients in the final stages of their long-term condition are to be adequately addressed (Fitzsimmons et al. 2007).

Although it is difficult to predict the prognosis for patients with a respiratory disease, one can consider lung function, frequency of exacerbations, loss of weight, other co-morbidities (such as heart failure) and the patients' requirement for long-term oxygen therapy. All these factors can help identify those patients who are entering the final year of life. Certainly, end-stage COPD should be suspected when a patient has very severe COPD, and the forced expiratory volume in 1 second is less than 30% of the predicted result (NICE 2015). When they score grade 4 or 5 on the MRC **dyspnoea** scale (PCRS 2015) and they are unresponsive to medical treatment, this is associated with a probable life expectancy of less than 6–12 months (NICE 2015). For these palliative care patients, the aim is to relieve symptoms and improve their quality of life, linking primary and secondary care as necessary.

Management of breathlessness

Breathlessness (dyspnoea) means 'disordered breathing' (Renwick 2001) but is also used to describe the patient's sensation of uncomfortably laboured breathing or chest tightness (Uronis et al. 2008). Chronic/persistent breathlessness is a common sign of COPD; and management of chronic breathlessness is a key aspect of treating and managing COPD, which is often treated using pharmacological methods (GOLD 2016). It is also helpful to understand breathlessness from a patient's perspective, as it can make them feel anxious and alone (Krishnasamy et al. 2001). These patients have often experienced breathlessness for many years, as it slowly worsens with time (Gysels & Higginson 2011). By the time they seek help, their difficulty in breathing is therefore a significant problem. A treatment programme that includes management strategies for dyspnoea has been found to produce a significant improvement in exercise tolerance and health-related well-being, reducing anxiety or depression (Sassi-Dambron 1995).

Although oxygen therapy is a treatment for **hypoxaemia** (not breathlessness), there are instances when it is used for chronic breathlessness – especially in palliative care (British Thoracic Society 2015).

There are also additional services available, such as the breathlessness support service integrated respiratory medicine, palliative care, physiotherapy, and occupational therapy for patients with advanced conditions and refractory breathlessness (Higginson *et al.* 2014). The service is responding to calls for earlier integration of palliative care, and evidence shows that patients using this service have an improvement in confidence, function, and control over their breathlessness.

Summary

Respiratory disease requires a personalised approach to medicine, which shifts from the disease to medicine that is focused on being predictive, preventative, personalised and participatory. We can argue that nurses have always used this integral and holistic approach. Wherever patients receive care, we know it should be patient-centred and holistic in nature. The core elements of palliative care should include aligning treatment with a patient's goals and management of their symptoms. Successful examples of these services have been mentioned, such as the breathlessness support service, and the British Thoracic Society provides very helpful information in these guidelines: https://www.brit-thoracic.org.uk/document-library/clinical-information/copd/copd-guidelines/bts-intermediate-care-hospital-at-home-for-copd-guideline/

References

Addington-Hall, J. (2002). Research sensitivities to palliative care patients. *European Journal of Cancer Care England.* **11**, 220–224.

Audit Commission (2000). *The way to go home: rehabilitation and remedial services for older people.* London: Audit Commission.

British Thoracic Society (BTS) (2015). *Guidelines for oxygen use in adults in healthcare and emergency settings.* https://www.brit-thoracic.org.uk/document-library/clinical-information/oxygen/emergency-oxygen-guideline-20 (Accessed 5.12.2016)

Curtis, J.R. (2008). Palliative and end-of-life care for patients with severe COPD. *European Respiratory Journal.* **32**(3), 796-803.

Davies, L., Wilkinson, M. & Bonner, S. (2000). 'Hospital at home' versus hospital care in patients with exacerbations of chronic obstructive pulmonary disease: prospective randomised controlled trial. *British Medical Journal.* **321**, 1265–1268.

Davison, A.G., Monaghan, M., Brown, D., Eraut, C.D., O'Brien, A., Paul, K. & Cubitt, L. (2006). Hospital at home for chronic obstructive pulmonary disease: an integrated hospital and community based generic intermediate care service for prevention and early discharge. *Chronic Respiratory Disease.* **3**(4), 181–185.

Department of Health (DH) (2001). *Intermediate Care.* HSC 2001/1: LAC (2001) 1. London: Stationery Office.

Department of Health. (DH) (2004). *The NHS plan. A plan for investment, a plan for reform.* London: Stationery Office.

Fitzsimons, D., Mullan, D., Wilson, J.S., Conway, B., Corcoran, B., Dempster, M. & MacMahon, J. (2007). The challenge of patients' unmet palliative care needs in the final stages of chronic illness. *Palliative Medicine.* **21**(4), 313–322.

Global Initiative for Chronic Obstructive Lung Disease (GOLD) (2016). *Global Strategy for Diagnosis, Management, and Prevention of COPD.* http://www.goldcopd.org/global-strategy-diagnosis-management-prevention-copd-2016/ (Accessed 3.12.2016).

Gore, J., Brophy, C. & Greenstone, M. (2000). How well do we care for patients with end stage chronic obstructive pulmonary disease (COPD)? A comparison of palliative care and quality of life in COPD and lung cancer. *British Medical Journal Thorax.* **55**, 1000–1006.

Gysels, M. & Higginson, I. (2011). The lived experience of breathlessness and its implications for care: a qualitative comparison in cancer, COPD, heart failure and MND. *BMC Palliative Care.* **10**, 15.

Hernandez, C., Casas, A., Escarrabill, J. et al. (2003). Home hospitalisation of exacerbated chronic obstructive pulmonary disease patients. *European Respiratory Journal.* **21**, 58–67.

Higginson, I. J., Bausewein, C., Reilly, C.C., Gao, W., Gysels, M. & Dzingina, M. & Moxham, J. (2014). An integrated palliative and respiratory care service for patients with advanced disease and refractory breathlessness: a randomised controlled trial. *The Lancet Respiratory Medicine.* **2**(12), 979–987.

Kent, J., Payne, C., Stewart, M. & Unell, J. (2002). *External evaluation of the Home Care Reablement Pilot Project.* Leicester: De Montfort University Centre for Group Care and Community Studies.

Krishnasamy, M., Corner, J., Bredin, M., Plant, H. & Bailey, C. (2001). Cancer nursing practice development: understanding breathlessness. *Journal of Clinical Nursing.* **10**(1), 103–108.

Melis, R., Rikkert, M., Parker, S. & Eijken, M. (2004). What is intermediate care? An international consensus on what constitutes intermediate care is needed. *British Medical Journal.* **329**(7462), 360–361.

Moon, J.T., McGlinn, T. et al. (2002). Patients' and carers' preferences in two models of care for acute exacerbations of COPD: results of a randomised controlled trial. *Thorax.* **257**, 167–171.

NICE (2015). *Chronic obstructive pulmonary disease.* http://cks.nice.org.uk/chronic-obstructive-pulmonary-disease (Accessed 5.12.2016).

Oliveira, J.C., Filho, F.S.L., Sampaio, L., Oliveira, A.C., Hirata, R., Costa, D., Donner, C. & Oliveira, L.V. (2011). Outpatient vs. home-based pulmonary rehabilitation in COPD: A randomized controlled trial. *European Respiratory Journal.* **38**(no pagination)

Primary Care Respiratory Society (PCRS) (2015). *The dyspnoea scale.* https://www.pcrs-uk.org/mrc-dyspnoea-scale (Accessed 5.12.2016).

Ram, F.S., Wedzicha, J.A. & Wright, J. (2004). Hospital at home for patients with acute exacerbations of chronic obstructive pulmonary disease: systematic review of evidence. *British Medical Journal.* **329**, 315.

Richards, S., Coast, J., Gunnell, J., Peters, T., Pounsford, J. & Darlow, M. (1998). Randomised controlled trial comparing effectiveness and acceptability of an early discharge, hospital at home scheme with acute hospital care. *British Medical Journal.* **316**, 1796.

Renwick, D. (2001) Breathlessness and quality of life in old age. *Age and Ageing.* **30**, 110–112.

Sassi-Dambron, D.E., Eakin, E.G., Ries, A.L. & Kaplan, R.M. (1995). Treatment of dyspnoea in COPD: a controlled clinical trial of dyspnoea management strategies. *CHEST Journal.* **107**(3), 724–729.

Skilbeck, J., Mott, L., Page, H., Smith, D., Hjelmeland-Ahmedzai, S. & Clark, D. (1998). Palliative care in chronic obstructive airways disease: a needs assessment. *Palliative Medicine.* **12**(4), 245–254.

Skwarska, E., Cohen, G. & Skwarski, K.M. (2000). Randomized controlled trial of supported discharge in patients with exacerbations of chronic obstructive pulmonary disease. *Thorax.* **55**, 907–912.

Sridhar, M., Taylor, R., Dawson, S., Roberts, N. & Partridge, M. (2008). Chronic obstructive pulmonary disease: A nurse led intermediate care package in patients who have been hospitalised with an acute exacerbation of chronic obstructive pulmonary disease. *Thorax.* **63**(3), 194–200.

Uronis, H.E., Currow, D.C., McCrory, D.C. *et al.* (2008). Oxygen for relief of dyspnoea in mildly- or non-hypoxaemic patients with cancer: a systematic review and meta-analysis. *British Journal of Cancer.* **98**, 294–299.

Glossary

2-Minute Walk Test (**2MWT**): measurement of endurance by assessing distance walked over 2 minutes.

accessory muscles: the sternomastoid, the scalenus anterior, medius and posterior, the pectoralis major and minor, the inferior fibres of serratus anterior and the latissimus dorsi.

acid-base balance: also known as homeostasis; refers to the balance between chemical acids and bases (also known as the body pH).

acidaemia: the state of low blood pH.

acidosis: the processes leading to a low pH.

adenovirus: a member of the *Adenoviridae* family of viruses. There are more than 40 types of adenovirus known to infect humans. They cause a range of diseases, from upper respiratory symptoms to gastroenteritis.

airway surface liquid (**ASL**): a very thin liquid layer that assists in removing particles from the lungs and airways.

alkalaemia: a state that occurs when the serum pH is higher than the normal level of 7.45.

alkalosis: a state that occurs due to the process of reducing the hydrogen ion concentration in arterial blood plasma.

allergen: a type of antigen that produces an abnormally immune response.

alpha 1-antitrypsin (**A1AT**): a protease inhibitor, so-called because it inhibits a wide variety of proteases and protects tissues from enzymes of inflammatory cells, especially neutrophil elastase.

alveoli: microscopic air sacs in the lungs where oxygen and carbon dioxide are exchanged.

amyotrophic lateral sclerosis (**ALS**): a progressive neurodegenerative disease that affects the neurological system, such as the nerve cells in the brain and spinal cord.

anaemia: a decrease in the total amount of red blood cells (RBCs) or haemoglobin in the blood.

angiotensin-converting enzyme (**ACE**): ACE inhibitors prevent an enzyme in the body from producing angiotensin II, which narrows the blood vessels and releases hormones that can raise the blood pressure.

anterior horn cell: there are two anterior horn cells – the anterior horn of lateral ventricle in the brain or the anterior horn of spinal cord.

antibody: a protein found in the bloodstream that is produced in response to, and counteracting, a specific antigen.

antigen: a toxin or any other foreign substance that induces an immune response in the body.

antigen presenting cell (**APC**): an APC, or accessory cell, displays an antigen complex with major histocompatibility complexes on their surfaces.

antineutrophil cytoplasmic antibody (**ANCA**): one of a group of auto-antibodies, which mainly consist of the IgG type.

aorta: the main artery of the body, which supplies oxygenated blood to the circulatory system.

arterial blood gas (**ABG**): this test measures the acidity (pH) and the levels of oxygen and carbon dioxide in the blood from an artery.

asbestosis: asbestosis is a chronic lung condition caused by prolonged exposure to asbestos.

ascites: a build-up of fluid between the two layers of the peritoneum.

asterixis: a tremor of the hand when the wrist is extended; also known as a flapping tremor, or liver flap.

asthma: a chronic inflammatory disease of the airways, characterised by variable and recurring symptoms of reversible airflow obstruction and bronchospasm.

atelectasis: the collapse of a lung, resulting in reduced or absent gas exchange.

atmospheric pressure: the pressure exerted by the weight of the atmosphere.

atopic eczema: the most common form of eczema.

atrial fibrillation: a condition where the heart rate is irregular and can be considerably higher than 100 beats per minute.

autosomal recessive disease: a type of disease created by two copies of an abnormal gene.

axilla: commonly known as the armpit.

baroreceptor: mechanoreceptor located in the carotid sinus and in the aortic arch; its role is to sense pressure changes in these areas.

barrel chest: a broad, deep chest shape found in people with a large ribcage, very round torso and a large lung capacity.

basophil: least common of the white blood cells called granulocytes.

bicarbonate buffering system: system in which carbon dioxide is dissolved in the blood, where it is taken up by red blood cells and converted to carbonic acid by carbonic anhydrase.

bicarbonate ion: a negatively charged ion, with the empirical formula HCO- 3; also known as a hydrogencarbonate ion.

body mass index (**BMI**): a measure that uses height and weight to work out if an individual's weight is healthy. To calculate the BMI, an adult's weight in kilograms is divided by their height in metres squared, e.g. a BMI of 25 means $25kg/m^2$. For most adults, an ideal BMI is between 18.5 and 24.9.

brainstem: stem-like part of the base of the brain that is connected to the spinal cord. It controls messages passed between the brain and the rest of the body, as well as basic body functions such as breathing, swallowing and heart rate.

bronchi: the main passageways into the lungs. When someone breathes in through their nose or mouth, the air travels into the larynx and then the trachea, which carries the air to the left and right bronchus, from where it passes into the lungs.

bronchiectasis: a long-term condition in which the airways of the lungs become abnormally widened, leading to a build-up of excess mucus that can make the lungs more vulnerable to infection.

bronchiolitis: a common lower respiratory tract infection that affects babies and young children under two years old.

bronchogram: a tubular outline of an airway made visible by filling of the surrounding alveoli by fluid or inflammatory exudates.

bronchophony: abnormal transmission of sounds from the lungs or bronchi, detected by auscultation.

bronchoscopic alveolar lavage (**BAL**): a diagnostic procedure in which lavage fluid is introduced to the terminal bronchioles and then recollected for analysis to examine cells, inhaled particles, infectious organisms or fluid constituents.

bronchoscopy: a procedure in which a hollow, flexible tube called a bronchoscope is inserted into the airways through the nose or mouth in order to view the tracheobronchial tree.

bronchospasm: a sudden constriction of the muscles in the walls of the bronchioles.

C6: the sixth cervical (neck) vertebra from the top.

candida: a yeast-like parasitic fungus that can sometimes cause thrush.

capillary: any of the fine branching blood vessels that form a network between the arterioles and venules.

carina of trachea: the ridge separating the openings of the right and left main bronchi where they join the trachea.

carotid artery: a major blood vessel in the neck that supplies blood to the brain, neck and face. There are two carotid arteries, one on the right and one on the left.

catalyse: to cause or accelerate a chemical reaction.

CD4+ cell: a cluster of 4 differentiation and a glycoprotein found on the surface of immune cells such as T helper cells, monocytes, macrophages and dendritic cells.

CD8 cell: a cluster of 8 differentiation and a transmembrane glycoprotein that serves as a co-receptor for the T cell receptor (TCR).

chemoreceptor: a sensory cell or organ that responds to chemical stimuli.

Cheyne Stokes breathing: a cyclical pattern of breathing in which movement gradually decreases to a complete stop and then returns to normal. It occurs in various medical conditions, and at high altitudes.

chronic obstructive pulmonary disorder (**COPD**): a lung disease in which the lung airflow is chronically obstructed; this interferes with normal breathing and is not fully reversible.

Churg-Strauss syndrome: a rare autoimmune condition that causes inflammation of small and medium-sized blood vessels (vasculitis) in people with a history of airway allergic hypersensitivity.

cilia: minute hairlike organelles that line the surface of certain cells and beat rhythmically, providing movement.

clavicle: commonly known as the collarbone.

collagen: the main structural protein found in animal connective tissue.

computed tomography (**CT**) scanning: a type of X-ray that can reveal anatomical details of internal organs that cannot be seen in conventional X-rays.

conjunctiva: the mucous membrane that covers the front of the eye and lines the inside of the eyelids.

coronavirus: one of a group of ribonucleic acid (RNA) viruses that cause various diseases in humans and other animals.

coryza: inflammation of the mucous membrane in the nose, often caused by a cold or by hay fever.

C-reactive protein (**CRP**): one of the plasma proteins whose plasma concentrations increase or decrease by 25% or more during inflammatory disorders.

crepitation: a dry, crackling sound or sensation.

cricoid cartilage: a complete ring of cartilage around the trachea, at the level of the C6 vertebra.

croup: inflammation of the larynx and trachea in children, associated with infection and breathing difficulties.

CURB-65: a simple scoring system that assigns 1 point for each of 5 clinical features (confusion status, urea level, respiratory rate, blood pressure, and age); it can be used to predict mortality in pneumonia and other infections.

cyanosis: a bluish discoloration of the skin due to poor circulation or inadequate oxygenation of the blood.

cystic fibrosis: an inherited condition in which the lungs and digestive system can become clogged with thick, sticky mucus.

cytomegalovirus: a kind of herpes virus that usually produces very mild symptoms but may cause severe neurological damage in newborn babies or people with weakened immune systems.

dendritic cell: an antigen-presenting cell (also known as an accessory cell) of the mammalian immune system. Its main function is to process antigen material and present it on the cell surface to the T cells of the immune system.

diabetic ketoacidosis: a serious complication of diabetes that occurs when the body produces high levels of blood acids called ketones. The condition develops when the body is unable to produce enough insulin.

diphtheria: an acute infectious disease caused by *Corynebacterium diphtheriae*, and characterised by the formation of a false membrane on the lining of the mucous membrane of the throat and other respiratory passages, causing difficulty in breathing, high fever and weakness.

duodenum: the first part of the small intestine immediately beyond the stomach, leading to the jejunum.

dyskinesia: abnormality or impairment of voluntary movement, resulting in fragmented or jerky motions as in Parkinson's disease.

dyspepsia: painful, difficult, or disturbed digestion, which may be accompanied by symptoms such as nausea and vomiting, heartburn.

dysphonia: commonly known as hoarse voice. For voice to be classified as 'dysphonic', there must be abnormalities in one or more vocal parameters: pitch, loudness, quality or variability.

dyspnoea: shortness of breath; a subjective difficulty in breathing that usually occurs at high altitude or during extreme exertion; also associated with serious disease of the heart, airways or lungs.

eczema: a medical condition in which patches of skin become rough and inflamed, with blisters that cause itching and bleeding.

egophony: more resonant voice sounds heard when auscultating the lungs, often caused by lung consolidation and fibrosis.

elastase: a pancreatic enzyme that breaks down and digests elastin.

emphysema: a chronic lung disease caused by irreversible damage to the alveoli. With emphysema, damage to the alveoli results in air becoming trapped, causing them to expand and rupture.

empyema: an accumulation of pus in the pleural cavity that can develop when bacteria invade the pleural space, usually in cases of pneumonia; also known as pyothorax or purulent pleuritis.

encephalopathy: a general term describing a disease that affects the function or structure of the brain.

endocrine cell: specialised cells of the gastrointestinal tract or pancreas that secrete hormones directly into the blood circulation, to be carried to the target cells.

endocytosis: the process by which a cell takes in material from the outside by engulfing and fusing it with its plasma membrane.

enzyme: a protein molecule that acts as a catalyst, helping other organic molecules undergo chemical reactions with one another.

eosinophil: a specific type of white blood cell that protects the body against certain kinds of germs, mainly bacteria and parasites; eosinophils also trigger allergic reactions.

epiglottitis: a flap of cartilage behind the root of the tongue, which is depressed during swallowing to cover the opening of the windpipe.

epistaxis: medical term for nosebleed.

epithelial cell: one of the closely packed cells forming the epithelium (membranous tissue that covers the internal organs).

erythema nodosum: a skin disorder characterised by painful red nodules that mostly appear on the shins.

erythrocyte sedimentation rate (**ESR**): a measure of how many red blood cells settle in a tube of blood during 1 hour; used to detect and monitor inflammation in the body.

extrinsic allergic alveolitis: a widespread disease of the lungs, involving inflammation in both the small airways and the alveoli (air sacs). It is not dissimilar to asthma, but the latter involves the bronchi and bronchioles.

exudate: a mass of cells and fluid that has seeped out of blood vessels or an organ, especially in inflammation.

fibrocyte: an inactive connective tissue cell that is capable of forming collagen.

finger clubbing: a deformity of the finger or toe nails associated with a number of diseases, mostly of the heart and lungs.

forced expiratory volume in one second (**FEV1**): the volume of air that can be forced out in one second after taking a deep breath, an important measure of pulmonary function.

forced vital capacity (**FVC**): the amount of air that can be forcibly exhaled from the lungs after taking the deepest breath possible; this test is used to help determine diagnose lung diseases and determine their severity.

fremitus: a sensation felt by a hand placed on a part of the body (such as the chest) that vibrates during speech.

full blood count (**FBC**): a common blood test to check a person's general health or to screen for conditions such as anaemia; the number of red cells, white cells and platelets in the blood are assessed.

gastro-oesophageal reflux disease (**GORD**): a disease of the lower oesophagus and stomach, also known as acid reflux; involves inflammation and irritation of the lower oesophagus due to the reflux of food and gastric acid.

glaucoma: a condition of increased pressure within the eyeball, causing gradual loss of sight.

glossopharyngeal nerve: the ninth cranial nerve, which supplies the tongue, throat and one of the salivary glands. Problems with the glossopharyngeal nerve can lead to difficulties with tasting and swallowing.

goblet cell: a column-shaped cell found in the respiratory and intestinal tracts, which secretes the main component of mucus.

gram-positive bacteria: bacteria that give a positive result in the gram stain test. Gram-positive bacteria take up the crystal violet stain used in the test, and then appear purple-coloured when viewed through a microscope.

granuloma: a collection of immune cells formed when the immune system attempts to wall off substances it perceives as foreign but is unable to eliminate; typically produced in response to infection, inflammation, or the presence of a foreign substance.

haematocrit: the percentage of red blood cells in the blood; a test to determine the percentage of red blood cells in the blood.

haemoglobin (**Hb**): a substance in red blood cells that combines with and carries oxygen around the body, and gives blood its red colour.

haemoptysis: spitting up blood or blood-tinged sputum from the respiratory tract; occurs when tiny blood vessels that line the lung airways are broken; can be due to a minor infection or a life-threatening medical emergency.

haemothorax: a pleural effusion in which blood accumulates in the pleural cavity; the excess fluid can interfere with normal breathing by limiting the expansion of the lungs.

health-related quality of life (**HRQOL**): an individual's or a group's perceived physical and mental health over time; used to measure the effects of chronic illness, treatments, and short- and long-term disabilities.

hepatitis: a disease characterised by inflammation of the liver; the condition can be self-limiting or can progress to fibrosis (scarring), cirrhosis or liver cancer.

hepatocyte: one of the chief functional cells of the liver, involved in synthesising protein.

hilar: relating to or affected by the hilus, which is positioned on the medial side of each lung, where the main bronchus, arteries and nerves enter the lung, and the main veins and lymphatic vessels leave it.

histamine: a compound released by cells in response to injury and in allergic and inflammatory reactions, causing contraction of smooth muscle and dilation of capillaries.

homeostasis: see acid-base balance.

Horner's syndrome: a relatively rare disorder caused by the disruption of a nerve pathway from the brain to the face and eye on one side of the body; typically results in a smaller pupil size, a drooping eyelid and decreased sweating on the affected side of the face.

hydrostatic pressure: the pressure exerted by a liquid.

hyoid bone: a horseshoe-shaped bone located in the anterior midline of the neck between the chin and the thyroid cartilage.

hypercapnia: a condition involving abnormally elevated CO_2 levels in the blood.

hyperglycaemia: having excess glucose in the bloodstream, often associated with diabetes mellitus.

hypokalaemia: having a deficiency of potassium in the bloodstream.

hyperkinesia: an increase in muscular activity that can result in excessive abnormal movements, excessive normal movements, or a combination of both.

hypertension: abnormally high blood pressure.

hypoesthesia: a reduced sense of touch or sensation, or a partial loss of sensitivity to sensory stimuli; in everyday speech, sometimes referred to as 'numbness'.

hypotension: abnormally low blood pressure.

hypoxaemia: abnormally low concentration of oxygen in the blood.

hypoxia: deficiency in the amount of oxygen reaching the tissues.

idiopathic pulmonary fibrosis: a condition in which the lungs become scarred and breathing becomes increasingly difficult.

immunoglobulin E: antibodies produced by the immune system. In an allergic individual, the immune system overreacts to an allergen by producing antibodies called immunoglobulin E (IgE). These antibodies travel to cells that release chemicals, causing an allergic reaction.

inhaled corticosteroid (IHC): anti-inflammatory asthma medication, taken using an inhaler.

interleukin: one of various small proteins, usually produced by white blood cells, which regulate many aspects of inflammation and the immune response, including stimulating the production of white blood cells and platelets.

intrathoracic pressure: pressure within the pleural cavity.

jaundice: a medical condition causing yellowing of the skin or whites of the eyes, resulting from excessive bilirubin pigment and typically caused by obstruction of the bile duct, by liver disease, or by excessive breakdown of red blood cells.

jugular venous pressure (JVP): blood pressure in the jugular vein.

Kussmaul breathing: rapid, deep and laboured breathing that is characteristic of patients with acidosis (excess acidity of tissues); often seen with acidosis of diabetes mellitus that is seriously out of control.

kyphoscoliosis: a deformity of the spine characterised by abnormal curvature of the vertebral column in two planes (coronal and sagittal); a combination of kyphosis and scoliosis.

kyphosis: excessive outward curvature of the spine, causing hunching of the back.

lactate dehydrogenase (LDH): an enzyme that the body uses when turning sugar into energy for the cells to use. LDH is found in many of the body's tissues and organs, including the muscles, liver, heart, pancreas, kidneys, brain and blood cells.

laryngeal stridor: a high-pitched breath sound resulting from turbulent air flow in the larynx.

laryngomalacia: a condition found in children when the soft, immature cartilage of the upper larynx collapses inward during inhalation, causing airway obstruction and stridor.

laryngopharynx: the lower part of the pharynx.

larynx: the muscular and cartilaginous-lined membrane of the trachea.

long-acting beta agonists (**LABA**): a type of long-acting bronchodilator.

long-acting muscarinic antagonist (**LAMA**): anticholinergic agent that blocks the activity of the muscarinic acetylcholine receptor and causes bronchodilation of the airways. It is called 'long acting' because it acts over 24 hours and the medication is used once a day. An example of this type of medication is tiotropium.

lumbar vertebrae: the five vertebrae between the rib cage and the pelvis that help support the weight of the body and allow movement to occur.

lumen: the internal space within a tubular structure such as an artery or vein.

lungs: a pair of organs found within the ribcage; they are elastic sacs with branching passages into which we inhale air so that oxygen can pass into the blood and carbon dioxide can be removed.

lung fibrosis: a medical condition in which the lung tissue becomes thickened, stiff and scarred over a period of time; also known as pulmonary fibrosis.

lymphadenopathy: a disease of the lymph nodes in which they are abnormal in size, number and shape.

lymphatic system: the network of tissues and organs that helps the body get rid of toxins and waste. It transports the lymph fluid, which contains white blood cells, throughout the body.

lymphocyte: a type of white blood cell known as a natural killer cell (NK cell). This is the main type of cell found in lymph system.

lymphoma: a form of blood cell tumour that develops from the specific white blood cell lymphocytes.

lysis: the process of dissolution or destruction of cells by lysins.

macrophage: a type of white blood cell that is part of the immune system. They engulf and digest cellular debris and foreign particles.

major histocompatibility complex (**MHC**): a group of genes that produce the code for proteins found on the surfaces of cells and enable the immune system to recognise foreign substances.

mean cell haemoglobin (**MCH**): the average mass of haemoglobin per red blood cell in any sample of blood.

mean corpuscular volume (**MCV**): the average volume of red blood cells.

mechanoreceptor: a receptor that picks up sensory information and responds to mechanical pressure or distortion.

mediastinum: the membranous partition between two body cavities seen between the lungs.

medulla oblongata: an anatomical term for the continuation of the spinal cord within the skull. It forms the lowest part of the brainstem and the control centre for the heart and lungs.

Meig syndrome: the triad of ascites, pleural effusion and a benign ovarian tumour.

mesenchymal cell: multipotent stromal cells that can differentiate into a variety of different cell types; also known as stem cells.

mesothelioma: a type of cancer that affects the lining of the lungs (pleural mesothelioma) but it can also affect the lining of the peritoneum, heart or testicles.

mitral stenosis: a narrowing of the mitral valve in the heart.

monocyte: one of the largest type of white blood cell, or leukocyte.

mucociliary escalator: a major barrier against infection. Microorganisms are caught in the sticky mucus in the airways and are then pushed upward towards the throat to be coughed up.

myalgia: muscle pain, which is a symptom of many diseases and disorders.

myasthenia gravis: a neurological disorder that results in muscle weakness and a lack of muscle strength.

myocarditis: a medical condition that causes inflammation and damage to the heart muscle.

myopathy: a muscular disease in which the muscle fibres do not work effectively, resulting in muscular weakness.

nasal cavity: the large air filled space above and behind the nose in the middle of the face; also known as the fossa.

nasopharynx: the upper part of the throat behind the nose and a part of the pharynx.

nephrotic syndrome: a condition that causes the kidneys to leak large amounts of protein into the urine.

neuron: an electrically excitable cell that processes and transmits information through electrical and chemical signals.

neutrophil: the most abundant type of granulocyte or white blood cell. Neutrophils have an important role in the innate immune system.

oedema: a condition in which fluid retention occurs in the surrounding tissue.

oesophagus: the organ through which food passes, aided by peristalsis, from the pharynx to the stomach.

oncotic pressure: a form of pressure exerted by proteins (such as albumin) in the blood vessel's plasma.

oropharynx: the middle part of the pharynx behind the mouth.

otitis media: an inflammatory disease of the middle ear.

packed cell volume (**PCV**): volume of packed red cells (VPRC), erythrocyte volume fraction; also known as haematocrit.

paraesthesia: abnormal sensations (such as tingling, tickling, pricking, numbness or burning) due to compression or damage to the nerve endings.

parenchyma: the functional tissue lining of an organ.

pathogen: microorganisms that cause disease such as bacteria.

peak expiratory rate (**peak flow**): a test that measures how fast a person can exhale (breathe out). This test checks lung functioning, and is often used for patients who have asthma.

pectus carinatum: a medical condition, also known as pigeon chest, characterised by a protrusion of the sternum and ribs.

pectus excavatum: a medical condition also known as sunken or funnel chest. It is a congenital chest wall deformity where several ribs and the sternum grow abnormally, causing a concave (caved-in) appearance in the anterior chest wall.

pericarditis: a condition caused by inflammation of the pericardium.

pertussis: a highly contagious respiratory disease caused by the bacterium Bordetella pertussis; commonly known as whooping cough.

phagocyte: cell found within the immune system that protects the body by ingesting harmful foreign particles, bacteria and dead or dying cells.

phagocytosis: the process by which phagocytes ingest or engulf other cells or particles within the body.

pharyngitis: inflammation of the pharynx, mainly due to a viral or bacterial infection.

pharynx: the anatomical part of the throat that is behind the mouth and nasal cavity and above the oesophagus and the larynx.

phenotyping: the process of predicting an organism's phenotype using information from their DNA sequencing; also known as DNA phenotyping.

phosphorylation: an effective way of regulating proteins.

pleura: the serous membrane which folds back onto itself to form a two-layered membranous pleural sac.

pleural effusion: occurs when excess fluid accumulates in the pleural cavity.

pleural rub: a noise that may be present in some patients with pleurisy and other conditions affecting the chest cavity.

pleural space: the thin fluid-filled space between the two pulmonary pleurae of each lung; also known as the pleural cavity.

pneumoconiosis: a restrictive lung disease caused by the caused by the inhalation of dust particles, such as coal dust or asbestos fibres.

pneumonia: a condition of the lung in which the alveoli (microscopic air sacs) become inflamed; mainly caused by various bacterial or viral infections.

pneumothorax: a condition in which there is an abnormal collection of air in the pleural space that causes movement of the lung from the chest wall.

polycythaemia: a disease in which the proportion of blood volume that is occupied by red blood cells increases.

pons: a part of the brainstem found between the midbrain (above) and the medulla oblongata (below) and in front of the cerebellum.

psychogenic breathlessness: dyspnoea or breathlessness due to stress and anxiety; characterised by irregular breathing and deep sighs.

ptosis: a drooping of the upper eyelid.

pulmonary embolism: a blockage of an artery in the lungs by a substance that has migrated from elsewhere in the body through the bloodstream (embolism).

pulmonary hypertension: elevated blood pressure within the pulmonary arteries.

pulse oximetry: a non-invasive test to monitoring a person's oxygen saturation (SO_2).

pyrexia: a rise in the body's normal core temperature.

radial artery: the main artery of the lateral aspect of the forearm.

radioallergosorbent (RAST) testing: a blood test that uses a radioimmunoassay test to detect IgE antibodies and then to determine the substances a subject is allergic to.

Reye's syndrome: a rare but serious condition that can lead to swelling in the liver and brain. It can occur in children once they have been exposed to chicken pox or flu.

rhinitis: irritation and inflammation of the nasal passages and mucosa.

rhinovirus: there are over 100 different rhinoviruses which cause most common colds. They are a genus within the *Picornaviridae* family of viruses.

rhonchi: low-pitched wheezes that are continuous during inspiratory and expiratory breaths. These low-pitched adventitious lung sounds are similar to wheezes.

sarcoidosis: a disease that causes abnormal collections of inflammatory cells that form lumps known as granulomas in the lungs, skin or lymph nodes.

sensory receptor: a sensory nerve ending that responds to a stimulus in the internal or external environment.

short-acting beta2 agonist (SABA): a type of medication that is commonly used for immediate relief of asthma symptoms. An example is salbutamol.

short-acting muscarinic antagonist (SAMA): a type of anticholinergic agent that blocks the activity of the muscarinic acetylcholine receptor and causes bronchodilation of the airways. It is short-acting medication. An example is ipratropium.

sinusitis: infection of the air-filled cavities or sinuses found at the front of the face.

soft palate: as the name suggests, this is the soft tissue at the back of the roof of the mouth; also known as the velum or muscular palate.

spirometry: lung function tests used to diagnose and monitor obstructive or restrictive respiratory disease.

sputum: the mixture of saliva and mucus that is coughed up from the respiratory tract. Medical conditions can create a change in colour, odour and consistency, which can be used as an aid to diagnosis.

stenosis: abnormal narrowing of a canal.

sternal notch: the large, visible dip between the neck and the collarbone; also known as the jugular notch.

sternum: the long flat bone shaped like a necktie, located in the centre of the chest; also known as the breastbone.

stridor: the harsh or grating sound made from an obstruction of the windpipe or larynx.

subphrenic abscess: this occurs when there is an accumulation of infected fluid between the diaphragm, liver and spleen.

surfactant: a compound that lowers the surface tension (or interfacial tension) between two liquids or between a liquid and a solid. It is found in the lungs.

systemic lupus erythematosus (SLE): an autoimmune disease in which the body's immune system mistakenly attacks healthy tissue in many parts of the body. The disease can affect every physical system so the symptoms are extensive.

tachycardia: also known as tachyarrhythmia; the name given when the heart rate exceeds the normal resting rate. In adults, this is generally accepted as 100 beats per minute.

tachypnoea: the name given to a respiratory rate that is greater than 20 breaths per minute.

TCR-CD3 complex: consists of a protein with a cluster of differentiation 3 T-cell co-receptors and helps to activate the cytotoxic T-cell.

Th1 response +Th2 response: Th1 and Th2 are subsets of the helper T lymphocytes expressing CD4; they are regarded as the most prolific cytokine producers.

thyrotoxicosis: a hereditary disease causing hyperthyroidism; also known as Graves-Basedow disease or Graves' disease.

T-lymphocyte: a member of the lymphocyte family; produced in the thymus and found circulating in the blood and lymph system. T-lymphocytes regulate the immune system's response to infected or malignant cells.

trachea: also known as the windpipe, this is the large membranous tube that extends from the larynx to the bronchial tubes. It is reinforced by rings of cartilage to keep it patent in order to convey air to and from the lungs.

tracheal tug: an assessment sign in which the trachea moves in a downward movement; also known as Oliver's sign.

tracheomalacia: a medical condition in which the tracheal support cartilage is so soft that the trachea partly collapses, especially during increased airflow.

transudate effusion: effusion caused by fluid leaking into the pleural space.

transverse myelitis: a neurological condition in which the nerve fibres become inflamed. This results in decreased electrical conductivity in the central nervous system.

tuberculosis: an infectious disease caused by the bacterium Mycobacterium tuberculosis, which generally affects the lungs, but can also affect other parts of the body.

vagal nerve: the tenth cranial nerve, which interfaces with parasympathetic control of the heart, lungs and digestive tract; also called the pneumogastric nerve.

vesicular breathing: lower-pitched, rustling sounds with higher intensity, heard during inspiration. During expiration, the sound intensity can quickly fade.

vocal resonance: the process by which the basic sound of phonation is enhanced through the air-filled cavities through which it passes.

whispering pectoriloquy: the increased loudness of whispering heard during auscultation with a stethoscope on the lung fields.

xiphisternal joint: a location near the bottom of the sternum, where the body of the sternum and the xiphoid process meet, in line with the T9 vertebra.

Index

'3 questions' screening tool 69

accessory muscles 4
acidaemia 8
acid-base balance 40
acidosis 8, 30
action plan 89, 90
air flow 3
airflow obstruction, severity of 43
airways 2
alkalaemia 8
alkalosis 8
allergen avoidance 70
allergen testing 44
alpha-1 antitrypsin 38
alpha-1 antitrypsin (A1AT) deficiency 19,
    64, 65
alveoli 1, 2, 3
anatomical landmarks of the chest 29
antibiotics 101
antihistamines 100
arterial blood gas 40
asbestosis 75, 76
aspirin sensitivity and asthma 68
asthma 59, 60, 66–73
asthma aetiology 66
Asthma–Chronic Obstructive Pulmonary
    Disease Overlap Syndrome (ACOS)
    61
asthma diagnosis 67, 68
asthma in children 68
asthma management 69
asthma, pharmacological management
    of 70, 71
asthma triggers 72
auscultation 33

baroreceptors 8
beta-blockers 18
bicarbonate buffering system 8
blood gas analysis 40
blood tests 38
BODE method 45
body mass index 30
breastfeeding and asthma 70
breath sounds 33
breathing, control of 7
breathing mechanism 3
breathing patterns 32

breathlessness, management of 109, 110
breathlessness, types and causes of 23
bronchi 1, 2
bronchial thermaplasty 102
bronchiectasis 76, 77, 78
bronchioles 1
bronchitis, acute 47

carina 2
cellular respiration 6
chemoreceptors 8
chest and neck, inspection of 31
chest expansion, assessment of 32
chest x-rays 41, 42
Cheyne Stokes breathing 30, 32
cholinesterase inhibitors 100
COPD 59–64, 86
COPD diagnosis 61, 62
COPD, management of 62
cough 21
cough, causes of 22
CRB65 score 51
cricoid cartilage 2
cromolyn 98
CURB65 score 51
cystic fibrosis 3, 18

daily dosing 89
data, subjective v. objective 16
diaphragm 4
dosing regimes 89

eczema 30
end of life care 109
erythema nodosum 30
exercise testing 44

face, inspection of 31
forced vital capacity 43
fremitus 32
full blood count 39

gas transfer testing 43
gas transport 9
genetic screening 65
genogram 19
goblet cells 2

haematocrit 39
haemoglobin 9, 39
haemoptysis 22

haemothorax 54
hands, inspection of 30, 31
history taking 15–21
home-based care 108
HOPE questionnaire 20
hypercapnia 8, 55
hyperventilation syndrome (HVS) 79, 80

idiopathic pulmonary fibrosis 74
immune response 10, 11
immunisation 102
influenza 48, 49
inhaled corticosteroids (IHCs) 98
inhaled medication 95
inhaler technique 85, 86
intercostal muscles 4
intermediate care 107, 108

jugular venous pressure 31

Kussmaul breathing 32

laryngeal cartilage 2
larynx 1, 2
leukotriene receptor antagonists 99
long-acting beta agonists (LABAs) 96, 97
lung cancer 78, 79
lung cancer management 79
lung function tests 42
lung volume reduction surgery (LVRS)
    102
lungs 1, 3, 5

mechanoreceptors 7
medication adherence 85, 86, 87
medication review 85
mesothelioma 76
MRC breathless scale 16
mucolytics 98
muscarinic antagonists 97

nasal cavity 1
nebuliser therapy 101, 102
non-adherence to medication 87
non-small cell lung cancer (NSCLC) 78, 79
NSAIDs 18

obstructive diseases 59
occupational asthma 68
oral bronchodilators 99, 100
oxygen therapy 64, 110
oxygen transportation 9

PAINT mnemonic 73, 74
palliative care 109
patient education 88
peak expiratory rate 42
pectoriloquy 34, 35
percussion 32
pharmacological therapies for COPD 63
pharmacology and respiratory disease 95–103
pharynx 1, 2
phosphodiesterase-4 inhibitors 98
physical assessment 29–35
pleura 1
pleural effusion 52, 53, 54
pneumonia 50, 51
pneumothorax 54, 55
polycythaemia 39
PQRST acronym 17
pulmonary rehabilitation 63
pulse 30

respiration, local control of 7
respiration, process of 6

respiratory assessment 15–25
respiratory centre in the brain 7
respiratory disease, acute presentations of 47–56
respiratory disease, cardinal signs of 21, 22, 23
respiratory diseases, chronic 59–81
respiratory failure 55, 56
respiratory muscles 4, 5
respiratory pattern 30
respiratory rate 30
respiratory rate, normal 7
respiratory system, anatomy and physiology of 1–12
respiratory system, defence of 10
respiratory system, function of 6
restrictive lung disease 73
Reye's syndrome 49

sarcoidosis 75
self-management 85–91
self-management and adherence 88
short-acting beta2 agonists (SABAs) 95, 96

skin 30
small cell lung cancer 78
smoking cessation 62, 78
spiritual beliefs 20
spirometry 42, 43
sputum cultures 40, 41
sputum production 22
sternal notch 2
stridor 32
surgery 102

tests for respiratory conditions 37, 38
trachea 1, 31
tracheomalacia 2
treatment adherence 86
tuberculosis 51, 52

vocal resonance 34

wheeze 22
work-related diseases 20